BALANCED AND WHOLE

21 DAY
JUMPSTART PROGRAM
FOR WEIGHT LOSS AND WELLNESS

JULIE COHEN, CHHC — BILL MCHUGH, MS, CPT

WELLNESS WORKS

Morristown, NJ

Wellness Works
18 Herms Place
Morristown, NJ 07960

Book layout by The Book Makers
Illustrations by Katie Emmitt
Julie Cohen's photo by Bart Gorin, Bart Gorin Photography
Bill McHugh's photo by Memories of Me Too Photography

Library of Congress Control Number: 2015943080

Dirty Dozen Plus™ and Clean 15™ are trademarks of The Environmental Working
    Group.
Finding Nemo© is a copyright of Disney/Pixar
Star Wars™ and character names are registered trademarks and copyright of
    Lucasfilm Ltd.
Eat Well Guide® is a registered trademark of Grace Communications Foundation
Ezekiel 4:9® is a registered trademark of Food For Life® Baking Company
Amore® is a registered trademark of PANOS™ Brands.
Tabasco® is a registered trademark of the McIlhenny Company
Cholula® is a registered trademark of Salsas de Jalisco Cacu, S.A. de C.V.
Mediterranean Organic ™ is a trademark of Mediterranean Organic
Post-it® is a registered trademark of 3M Corporation.
TRX® is a registered trademark of Fitness Anywhere, LLC.
Muir Glen® is a registered trademark of Small Planet Foods.
Vitamix® is a registered trademark of the Vita-Mix Corporation.
Thin Mints® is a registered trademark of Girl Scouts of the USA.

Ordering Information:
Quantity sales. Special discounts are available on quantity purchases by corporations, associations, and others. For details, contact the "Special Sales Department" at the address above.

Balanced and Whole / Julie Cohen and Bill McHugh—1st ed.
ISBN print 978-0-9963760-0-6
ISBN ebook 978-0-9963760-1-3

Thank you to:

*My dad, Frank Giraldi, for teaching me by example
that we are each in charge of our own health,*

*My mom, Mary Giraldi, for teaching me that
love is the most important main ingredient, and*

*My husband, Phil Cohen, for being
the only main ingredient I've ever needed.*

— Julie Cohen

*In memory and thanksgiving to my mom, Mary Valentine McHugh,
whose giving, adventurous and loving heart showed us how to live whole with
good nutrition and an active body to enjoy a passionate and purposeful life.*

*My dad, who by example and quiet words of wisdom,
taught balance by keeping a positive and happy attitude and
to be appreciative for all that we have.*

*My wife Kathy, whose constant love and support has been
the wind beneath my wings and key to my health and happiness.*

— Billy McHugh

*A Big Shout Out to Dave Walters and his awesome crew at Smart World
of Morristown, where we held many meetings to finely grind out and
filter through the material for this book....Smart World serves delicious,
sustainably harvested coffee with a healthy side of community!*

— Julie & Billy

Contents

Important Alerts

WE RECOMMEND THAT YOU CONSULT your physician and have a thorough physical exam and complete blood work prior to initiating the Balanced and Whole 21-day Jumpstart Program. This program involves exercises that require physical exertion that, while they may be extremely beneficial, may also be stressful to your system. You should be cleared by your physician before initiating this program, especially those who are over 40 years old, smoke, are on medication, have known heart disease, diabetes, high cholesterol, high blood pressure, obesity, anxiety, depression, sleep disorders or other illnesses, disease and conditions.

The Balanced and Whole 21-day food program is intended only for adults with no specific health or allergy concerns that may require medical supervision.

The advice and nutritional recommendations are not intended to diagnose, treat or cure in any manner whatsoever, any disease, condition or other physical or mental ailment of the human body. The authors are not engaged in rendering professional advice to the individual reader or in acting in the capacity of a doctor or licensed dietician-nutritionist.

Before making any changes to your diet, you should consult with your healthcare professionals, including, without limitation, your physician.

A word from Bill McHugh

"Health is a state of complete physical, mental and social well-being and not merely the absence of disease or infirmity".
– Preamble to the constitution of the World Health Organization

CONGRATULATIONS ON TAKING THE FIRST steps towards improving your health and well-being! We are very excited to assist you in a program that can have a very positive life-changing impact on you. The Balanced and Whole 21-Day Jumpstart Program is not an easy, quick-fix, short-term diet that you begin and then stop, falling back into old habits. This plan is rather a fresh, health-enhancing endeavor that is intended to set you up for long-term, permanent change!

Change is not easy, as we are a product of our habits and our habits are a result of our conditioned behaviors. We have been conditioned our entire lives to behave the way we do; therefore, in order to break these old conditioned patterns of behavior or "bad habits," we need more than just will power—we want to replace them with consistent, repetitive good habits.

I realize now how I formed some healthy habits as a child. Having grown up in a family with 9 other siblings was an adventure, to say the least. My folks had to be resourceful to feed 10 kids! As young children, we were fortunate that my parents got us involved in every component of planting a huge garden. We helped clear a large section of land in our backyard, dug up and removed the rocks, shoveled in healthy soil, planted the fruits and vegetables and then the best part—picked the harvest, a wide variety of fruits and veggies! I didn't realize at the time the many good behavioral benefits I was getting and how nutritionally fortunate I was, being able to walk out into this amazing garden in the morning and pick fresh strawberries to put in my cereal, or in the evening to get fresh fixings for a salad! I was conditioned daily by my parents and siblings to eat healthy and stay active at a young age and am now motivated to help you initiate healthy habits today! The good news is that you can start creating and changing habits at any age, and we are here to show you how to do this in 21 days!

Why 21 days?

By committing to this easy-to-follow, step-by-step exercise and nutrition plan for 21 days straight, your body will be going through many positive changes and you will be "jumpstarted" into feeling much better. As you lay down a solid whole-food eating and exercise foundation, you will gain momentum for continuing on a program for long term success.

While we realize that breaking long-term habits such as smoking cigarettes, changing sleep patterns and stopping late night snacking may take longer than 3 weeks, our focus is not as much on getting you to break old habits but rather to form new, healthier ones. It's easier to form a new habit than to break an old one. So our goal is to help you change some of your current behaviors by forming new, beneficial eating and exercising behaviors.

Although it is a challenge, 21 days is an achievable time frame. Three weeks gives you an ample amount of time to form a good healthy base upon which you can continue to build. To make it more manageable, we have broken the program down into three, bite-size weekly "portions" that are easy to digest. Julie and I are here to coach you through the 21-day process and have outlined easy-to-follow guidelines to keep you on track.

What do you want to get out of this program?

To help you succeed, you need to first ask yourself, why am I doing this program? What do I want to get out of this 21-day challenge? What do I want to change? What do I want to achieve? What are my personal health and fitness goals? Your first step then towards committing to change is to write down your desired goals. If you are serious about making positive change, you need to help make it tangible. Your first action or "exercise" then, towards actualizing your goals, is putting them down on paper.

This may seem trivial or basic, but it is extremely important. Are you looking to lose weight? Do you want to eat healthier, "cleaner," less sugar, more fruits and vegetables? Do you want to tone up and boost your metabolism and increase bone density? Do you need to decrease your blood sugar, blood cholesterol, or blood pressure? Do you want more energy, to be less stressed, to sleep better, have less aches and pains, to slow the aging process or just feel better overall? Well, then, you must write it down! Stop immediately, flip to your Personal Goal Achievement Agreement on page 23 and take a few minutes to write down your short-term and long-term goals now!

Putting it all together...

Perhaps you have gone on various diets for weight loss or tried eating well for a while and fallen off the path. Maybe you worked out for a period of time and were frustrated by not getting the results you wanted or were side-tracked by "stuff" in life. It's easy to get distracted and discouraged. But be honest with yourself...have you actually combined both eating healthy and exercising consistently for any length of time? By combining both exercise and healthy eating, your results will be accelerated, your ability to stick to the program will be great and your overall feeling will be amazing! So for optimal health and well-being, you can't just eat well, and you can't just exercise—you have to balance your program by combining both.

Here is the good news: You don't have to exercise for hours every day and starve yourself to achieve great results! As a matter of fact, this program is designed for you to do just 30 minutes of exercise per day to reach your health and fitness goals! The key is staying consistent long enough to "get hooked" on feeling great! Our plan helps you move past the challenging startup phase and gain traction for continued results.

Being Balanced & Whole…what's it really all about?

Are you functioning at your fullest potential? Our long term goal for you is to not only be eating whole foods and exercising but also living whole. Living whole as a person means being balanced and well in every area of your life: mentally, physically and spiritually. Will your health be good in the future? Do you want to be a victim of inactivity and premature aging? As you age, what is your quality of life going to be? Are you going to subject yourself to taking handfuls of medication (are you now)? Are you going to be self-sufficient? Will you be spending exorbitant amounts of money on doctors, medicines and therapy aids? What is stopping you from being the absolute best you can be?

Following our jump start program for eating whole food and exercising regularly will help you establish the consistent pattern that you can continue and make part of your week. This 21-day period is a fresh beginning that you can continue to build upon each day to become "balanced and whole." The Balanced and Whole 21-Day Program will Jumpstart you NOW to feel well, think well, move well and get more out of life!

Ultimately, this book is a guide to help you start on the path of living happier with greater peace of mind. So don't just go through life passively, waiting for disease to set in. Rather set your goals high, "behave yourself" into being active and eating healthy and break through those barriers that have been holding you back and you will live life long, vibrant and well! Don't you deserve to live happy and fulfilled?

"We are what we repeatedly do. Excellence, therefore,
is not an act but a habit."
–Aristotle

A word from Julie Cohen

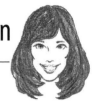

Food Magic

WHAT I'VE LEARNED FROM BEING a Health Counselor, above all else, is that there really is no one magic solution for everyone. No one perfect diet reflects what everyone should eat and will thrive on. The solution is one of trial and error; of discovering what fuel our body runs best on and feeding ourselves accordingly. Thriving is about accepting that our diet is dynamic. We will thrive on different diets at different periods in our lives, at different ages, different activity levels, different health challenges and even different philosophical phases. Food isn't supposed to be philosophical but it is. Food is about so much more than what we chew and swallow. It speaks to what we believe about the land, animal husbandry and our place in the puzzle. For many of us food is the most important way we connect to and nurture those we love, including ourselves!

When you think about it, the "magic part" exists in all areas of our lives, not just in food. In medicine, for example, how much the doctor cares or if the doctor holds the patient's hand makes a difference in patient outcomes. The magic part is critical but it's hard to measure so we avoid it.

If there's no one diet that's appropriate for all of us, how can one design a food program that will help many different people? I don't believe one can, if the food program requires specific foods in specific quantities—that's a "diet" and we all know how well those work! We each need to use trial and error to determine the best foods and food combinations for our body; however, without any structure it's easy to become overwhelmed and not know how to begin.

This program offers a structure, a framework into which you can place your meal choices. It moves fast, getting you onto a whole food eating plan from the get-go, and requiring you to do the work of listening to your body. It provides "Meal Skeletons"—the "bones" of your daily eating. You fill in the skeleton with the foods you choose. This requires more decision making than following a specific "meal plan" or eating prepackaged, portioned food, but it provides you with the portion control skills that you need to continue past the 21 days of the program. Living in good health is all about your choices. Every day you are making food choices. You may be drifting through your food life, eating whatever you happen to bump into, but this too is a decision! You can't change everything in 21 days. What you can do is begin to break some of the not-so-healthy habits you have now and start forming new, healthier ones. How far you take them is up to you.

Are you game?

Try something different from what you are doing now for precisely 21 days. During the 21 days we'll try to get you to simply evaluate, to become an observer of your life and take some notes. At the end of the 21 days, assess where you want to go. Maybe you'll want to seek out some help; and yes, there are plenty of people who can help, but ultimately, we are each responsible for our own choices.

If you stick to the program, you'll begin to form healthier habits. When you do something for 21 days straight you are on your way to forming a habit. At the end of that time, you will know a little more than you did before and weigh a little less than you did before and hopefully, you will be hungry to keep going!

Who should use this program?

This program is designed for healthy adults who are overweight and don't currently have a regular exercise or fitness regimen. People who would like to undertake changes in a speedy manner—to jump in with both feet.

Jumping in with both feet can give you a push, the momentum you need to motivate yourself to keep going. Don't view this program as a diet; view it as a whole foods experiment. You'll discover how you feel eating only whole foods. You'll find out if your body releases weight eating this way. You'll learn which foods and food combinations work better for you. It only requires dedicating more time to planning and preparing your food while still embracing the convenience of prepared, frozen and canned whole foods. It will also help you make healthier choices when you are eating out. It's a 3-week, "How-to" guide that you can adapt to your lifestyle— you don't have to go for perfect, just go for good enough!

Calling all sugar addicts...

When it comes to sugar, many of us are addicted and don't even know it. And when it comes to sugar, I believe "cold turkey" is the best way to go. It is often only this way that you can experience both the drastic difference in the way you feel off sugar and the drastic difference in the way food tastes. A simple strawberry or a raisin may become the sweetest thing you've ever tasted...this is the magic of eating whole foods! Your taste buds, which have been hijacked by processed foods and very high levels of sweeteners, will start to transform. Plus, avoiding added sugars for 21 days straight will significantly curtail your sugar cravings.

Calling all Omnivores...

This program is designed for omnivores. I don't believe in eliminating or demonizing any one food group. Our diets have been based on various fads over the last many years. First we got rid of "bad" fat (or so we thought) going hog wild with "carbs," and now we've moved on to overdosing on "protein," nutrition's new darling.

Each of these dietary imbalances has had consequences; trans-fat has been implicated in heart disease and excessive consumption of sweeteners and carbohydrate-based foods are implicated in diabetes.

Time will tell us more about the effects of too much protein in our diet. This program eschews diet fads.

Quality counts

The quality of your food counts. Buy organic and local if you can, or consider buying organic for at least the produce that is highest in pesticide residues. The Environmental Working Group's (EWG) *Dirty Dozen Plus*™, http://www.ewg.org/foodnews/ is a list of the conventionally-grown fruits and vegetables containing the highest concentrations of pesticide residues. Typically, this list is updated annually and it specifies when there are differences between the same produce item grown domestically or imported. Food stores are required to display the country of origin on produce so this offers helpful information. The EWG also provides the Clean 15™, a list of produce lowest in pesticide residues, foods that you don't need to buy organic. Utilizing these resources will help you to spend your "Organic Dollars" wisely.

Since you're going to be eating a lot more produce in this program, you want it to be of the highest quality you can afford. Use the money you save from fewer trips to your favorite coffee shop for some "energy in a cup" and spend it on fresh organic vegetables and fruit!

Quality counts just as much for animal foods: meat, dairy, eggs and seafood. Buy organic, pasture-raised, grass-fed and free range, if possible. Animals raised in a healthy way, who themselves were fed a healthy diet and exercised, are healthier and are therefore a healthier choice for us. The same can be said for seafood that is wild caught. These foods aren't cheap and that may mean you'll eat less of them, and that's fine!

Set yourself up for success!

The most important action you can take to be successful in your 21-Day Jumpstart is to look over all the materials ahead of time, including the whole foods lists, sample meals and snacks (if you need ideas), and the weekly meal skeletons. If you can't eat dry cereal for breakfast anymore, what will you eat instead? Plan for it. Go shopping and buy what you plan to eat in Week One. You need to plan for all three of your meals and possible snacks.

List and shop for your food the weekend before you begin the 21-Day Jumpstart. Whether you plan to cook all your meals or do a mixture of cooking and "building," which you'll learn more about—you have to plan! Cleaning and cutting up enough vegetables on Sunday to get you through to Thursday ensures that you will have what you need to follow the program when your week gets busy. Buying frozen vegetables and prewashed leafy greens also saves time. Purge your sweets and processed foods and stock up on enough whole foods to allow you to try a few different breakfasts, lunches, and dinners. At the end of Week One, review your food diary and evaluate what's working well and what isn't.

Get your Joy On!

The "big" celebrations aren't what life is mostly about, it's about the joy underlying each day. Sometimes we don't notice this subtle joy until something happens to temporarily cause its absence. Ideally, we never receive such a wakeup call. Being balanced means being more aware of the joy in our lives...if most of your joy has been coming from food, how are you going to fill that void? What else makes you joyful?

Most of my clients feel better when they start making a daily gratitude list; thinking of 5 small things they are grateful for each day. Things like a particularly positive interaction your kids had with each other, getting a big smile from someone, or not getting a parking ticket even though your meter ran out, to name a few. This is a good way to focus on the positive parts of your day and, if you're extra cranky without your sugar, you're going to need it!

Manage expectations...

If you have unrealistic expectations about weight loss this is the time to challenge them...this program is flexible, in terms of calorie consumption. You'll find a lot of variability when you are using "Meal Skeletons," which allows you to choose foods that you like, as opposed to following a "diet." It also teaches you how to eat, in terms of portion sizes and food group proportions. These are the most important skills for healthy eating over the long haul.

Eating only whole foods for 21 days is challenging but doing so will give you a taste of what is involved in eating a mostly whole foods diet. If you continue reaching for a whole food, instead of one in a "wrapper," you are on your way to a lifetime of healthier eating.

Every good decision you repeatedly make increases the odds that you will make another good decision. String these food decisions together, day after day, and you build habits, and habits help take the pain out of decision making.

Whatever happens, just keep swimming!

In the movie *Finding Nemo©*, the "Head Injured Fish," as we call her in my house, is named Dory. Dory's philosophy on life is one I go back to often, "Just keep swimming." Some days, we make food choices that fall somewhere on the continuum between "missing the mark" and "going bananas." When this happens, don't beat yourself up about it or use it as an excuse to fall OFF the program; instead, channel your "Inner Dory" and just keep swimming!

Balance

By Karen D. Kedar

Befriend the many aspects of self:
Mind, body, soul, emotions.
All form a tapestry of beauty,
Handcrafted for you by God.
It is the landscape of your life, your true self.
Deny none their rightful place,
Strive for an equal balance of all the parts.

Collect your emotions.
Unbury your soul.
Honor your body.
Calm your mind.

Balance.
Center.
Journey forth with every part of you
In alignment.

The poem "Balance" is from <u>God Whispers: Stories of the Soul,</u>
<u>Lessons of the Heart</u> © 1999 by Karen D. Kedar.
Permission granted by Jewish Lights Publishing,
P.O. Box 237, Woodstock, VT 05091
www.jewishlights.com

Balanced and Whole
Week One Exercise

THE KEY PIECES TO THE "FEELING WHOLE" PUZZLE

MANY NEW AND EXCITING CHANGES will be happening to your body over the next 21 days as you begin to get in shape, especially if you have not been exercising for a while. The exercise portion of this program works because it is:

- Time efficient
- Convenient
- Affordable
- Easy to follow
- Safe to perform

This program will jumpstart your body to begin:

- Boosting your metabolism, promoting fat "burning"
- Increasing its energy
- Decreasing stress and tension
- Adding lean body tissue to firm and tone muscle
- Improving cardiovascular endurance
- Increasing bone density
- Enhancing flexibility
- Sleeping better

SET YOURSELF UP FOR ACHIEVEMENT!

Four Steps to Achievement:

plan purposefully
prepare prayerfully
proceed positively,
pursue persistently.

– William A. Ward

Adherence

Convenience is essential for adherence. Performing your exercise program at home saves you time, money and frustration. I designed the 21-Day Jumpstart Exercise Program to be time-efficient and created it as an easy-to-follow workout in the convenience of your home.

Putting it all together does require a plan. The exercise portion of this program is clearly laid out for you with straight-forward guidelines, three easy-to-follow weekly workouts with illustrations for each exercise, and workout sheets to log your results.

Here are 7 tips to set yourself up for success:

1. Write down your specific long-term and short-term goals and keep them visible—remind yourself where you want to go. As author and business coach Stephen Covey said, "Begin with the end in mind."

2. Plan your week in advance; record your daily workouts on your calendar, in your planner, or on your phone.

    My wife, Kathy, will attest to the fact that I can be a bit obsessed with goal setting and planning. But it works! Goal setting and planning helps to shift your desire from "I want to do this" to a more solid, real commitment of "I will do this."

3. Take "before" photos, tape measurements and weigh yourself (to get a real awareness of where you are).

4. Choose workout days and times that are realistic and you can stick to daily.

5. Start an exercise journal and jot down what you did that day and how you felt. A Food and Exercise journal page is provided after each week's food diary pages.

6. Start out low intensity; do not over-train or try to do too much too soon!

7. Treat yourself to some new sneakers or workout clothes—get psyched about starting!

> *Before beginning your exercise program, be sure to undergo a full physical and obtain consent from your physician. We recommend that you do a wellness exam including blood work with a full lipid profile, and a stress test, if warranted.*

EXERCISE GUIDELINES FOR SAFE AND EFFECTIVE RESULTS
"Strength Day" Guidelines

Below are your strength-training guidelines for maximum results.

➤ *See Appendix A for pictures and descriptions of all exercises.*

- **Warm up**: Always include a good warm-up (at least 5 minutes of rhythmic movement) before jumping into strength-training exercises. Good warm-up activities are walking, stepping, light calisthenics, biking, skipping rope and shadow boxing.

- **Train Safe**: Perform each strength exercise slowly (2 seconds in the up or positive motion, and 4 seconds on the lowering or negative phase), and move quickly to the next exercise with minimal rest between exercises.

- **Sets and Reps**: Perform one set, 15 to 20 repetitions of each exercise, and do not hold your breath. Breathe by exhaling on the positive, faster movement.

- **Exercise Modifications**: If you cannot perform pushups or achieve the plank from your toes, then modify these exercises from your knees.

  See pictures of these exercise modifications in Appendix A. You can also start from your toes and do as many reps as you can in good form and then "break it down" to finish your reps from your knees (i.e. 10 pushups from toes, 10 modified pushups from knees).

- When performing the resistance band exercises, if you cannot do at least 15 reps with the medium weight band, i.e. overhead press and bicep curl exercises, use the lightweight band.

- **Cool Down**: Take 5 minutes to stretch after each strength workout.

➤ *See Appendix B for pictures and descriptions of all stretches.*

- **Recovery:** Rest 48 hours between strength workouts to allow ample time for your muscles to recover for optimal toning and strength gains.

"Cardio Day" Guidelines

- **Heart Rate Monitoring:** For optimal fat burning and cardiovascular conditioning results and to know you are exercising at safe levels for your body, it's important to monitor your heart rate during all your exercise sessions. This is done by making sure you are training in your age-adjusted target heart rate zone (THR). This "zone" is determined by exercising at 55 to 85% of your estimated maximum heart rate, designated by upper (maximum) and lower (minimum) heart rate levels in beats per minute

(BPM). To know what your THR Zone is, refer to the Target Heart Rate chart in Appendix D.

- For an easy way to assure you are training in your Target Heart Rate Zone, I recommend you purchase a heart rate monitor watch so that you'll know what your heart rate is throughout your workouts.

- If you choose to check your "active heart rate" manually during exercise, do this by taking a 10-second pulse count on your radial artery. Palpate on the thumb side of your wrist with your pointer and index fingers for 10 seconds and multiply the number of beats you get by 6 to get beats per minute. Referring to the Heart Rate chart, at age 50 your 10-second pulse count target is 16-24 beats in a 10-second count.

- Check your pulse in the middle and towards the end of your exercise sessions to assure you're in the appropriate heart rate range. You want to be working hard enough to get a cardiovascular training effect, but not so hard as to go over your upper level heart rate.

- **Duration:** Start with 10 to 15 minutes of continuous aerobic exercise and add 2 minutes for each workout until you get to 30 minutes. So if you start at 12 minutes of walking, and add two minutes to each of your 3 cardio days per week, by the end of 21 days you will be at 30 minutes!

- **Pace It:** Always warm up gradually, easing into your cardiovascular exercises, and cool down with flexibility stretches.

➤ *Refer again to Appendix B for pictures and descriptions of stretches.*

EXERCISE INTENSITY

- Upon initiating your exercise program, you may experience some delayed onset muscle soreness, or **"DOMS."** Some minor muscle soreness is normal after your first couple of workouts as you "wake up" some dormant muscles. However, your muscle discomfort should be mild, just enough to indicate you've done something new with your body, and you shouldn't be so sore that you can't get out of bed in the morning or walk down the stairs!

- **Rate of Perceived Exertion:** Another way to gauge the intensity level that you should be exercising at is by using a chart called the Rate of Perceived Exertion Scale. Exercise between a 4 and an 8 intensity level; not too light but not overly strenuous.

➤ *See Appendix D for the RPE scale.*

THE BENEFITS OF STRETCHING

Just as a warm-up is imperative prior to a workout, stretching is important after each workout and provides several positive benefits for you. Stretching does not have to involve a huge time commitment, but stretching can end up giving you huge results! Here are just a few of the benefits you can expect from a regular stretching program.

Physical Benefits of Stretching:
- Increased flexibility and joint range of motion
- Improved blood circulation to various parts of the body
- Better posture and body alignment
- Reduced muscle tension and stress relief

Additional Gains Include:
- Increased energy levels (resulting from increased circulation).
- Allowing your body time to safely "cool off." This enables your heart rate and blood pressure to safely come down and return to resting levels.

- Preventing post workout or delayed onset muscle soreness "DOMS." Why be tight and in pain after exercise when it can be prevented with 5 to 10 minutes of stretching!

Mental Benefits of Stretching:

A good workout combined with a cool-down period after exercise, involving slow static stretching and deep relaxed breathing, will illicit the brain to release "feel good" chemicals such as endorphins and serotonin. These chemicals are released by your central nervous system. Endorphins make you feel exhilarated and happy and block feelings of pain. Serotonin is the chemical responsible for happiness, restful sleep, and a healthy appetite. Stretching is a way to relieve stress and anxiety. Slow, focused stretching can lower your blood pressure and breathing rate, which helps to release tension from your body and calm your brain.

Listed in Appendix B are recommended stretches with illustrations and descriptions. These stretches should be done at the end of every cardio and strength workout.

Stretching Guidelines

- Make sure you are fully warmed up prior to stretching.
- Hold your stretches for 30 to 60 seconds. Do not bounce. Bouncing as you stretch can cause injury to your muscles.
- Start your stretching from the lying down position after your abdominal exercises. Then proceed to follow the enclosed sequence and flow from lying to the kneeling position, to sitting and then to standing (see Appendix B).
- Focus on taking slow, deep breaths in through your nose and out through your mouth when doing your stretching.

Sleep and Rest

We would be remiss in writing a book on being Balanced and Whole without mentioning how important rest and sleep is for good health and optimal well-being!

Rest and Workout Recovery

The appropriate amount of sleep and rest between workouts is crucial for your body's ability to recover, your continued desire to stay motivated and consistent, and to maximize your overall results. After a strength workout, your body needs time to repair in order to build muscle. So for optimal muscle toning, it is crucial to **refrain from doing strength training exercises for 48 hours between strength workouts.** However, I encourage you to do cardiovascular exercise and stretching between your strength workouts, not just to burn more calories and accelerate weight loss, but also to aid in your strength workout recovery.

The Impact of Sleep Deprivation on your Health

The evidence from a growing body of research on the importance and positive impact of getting sufficient sleep keeps building. I have noticed a growing focus in the health and wellness industry on the significance of sleep for your physical and mental health. Lack of sleep can:
- Weaken your immune system
- Impair your memory and cognitive ability
- Decrease focus, reaction time and coordination
- Cause irritability, anxiety and depression

Even more, both the amount of and quality of your sleep influences hormone activity tied to your appetite and feelings of hunger and fullness. The latest research is revealing that sleep loss could increase the severity of age-related ailments such as hypertension, diabetes, obesity and dementia!

Tips for a Better Night's Sleep

- **Create a Sleep-conducive Environment:** Start with the right bedding. Invest in a good mattress and comfortable pillow. After all, we spend approximately a third of our life in bed! Maintain the right room temperature. Take notice if you sleep better with the room cooler or warmer. Make sure your bedroom blocks out any outside noise and light.

- **Make it a Ritual:** Establish regular bedtime habits. Go to bed the same time every night. Your body's chemicals and hormones gradually will learn to establish a pattern and that will trigger you to prepare for sleep if you follow a daily ritual.

- **Exercise Timing:** It is fine to exercise right after work to burn off the accumulated stress of the day. But avoid vigorous exercise close to bedtime. It is best to exercise in the morning or during the day. You want to start slowing your body down as the day goes on.

- **Food and Drink:** This program eliminates almost all added sugars and discourages any snacking after dinner, which may improve the quality of your sleep. If you need a little help unwinding and relaxing before bed, try a cup of chamomile tea. Chamomile is an herbal (caffeine free) tea that promotes relaxation and sleep. Be aware, however, that drinking any liquid right before bed may result in nighttime waking to use the bathroom. Whenever possible, avoid ingesting food and liquids two to three hours before bed.

Summary of the Benefits of a Good Night's Sleep

- Increased fat metabolism and weight loss
- Enhanced muscle recovery and strength gains
- Better mental concentration and memory
- Less muscle and joint aches and pains
- Decreased anxiety, irritability and depression
- Improved coordination and reaction time
- Enhanced immune system

EXERCISE PROGRAM SCHEDULE AT A GLANCE

Strength Days   Mon-Wed-Fri: 30 minutes of strength training
Cardio Days   Tues-Thurs-Sat: work up to 30 minutes of cardio
Recovery Day   Sunday: rest or stretch

Equipment:

To get started all you need is the following equipment:

- A large fitness ball—45 cm (under 5'5" tall), 55 cm (5'5" to 6' tall), or 65 cm (over 6' tall)
- Two or three exercise resistance bands with handles and door anchors. *It is important to align the resistance bands with the door anchor to be able to shut the door on the anchor for some of the exercises in this program.*
  - One light weight resistant band (usually green),
  - One medium weight resistant band (usually blue or purple).
  - If you have been strength training consistently for several months, you may want to also purchase a heavy weight exercise band (usually black).
- Your own body weight

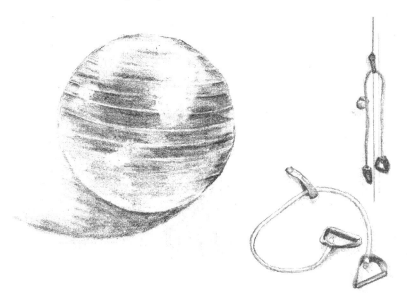

Personal Goal Achievement Agreement

I _____ do hereby commit to the activities
necessary to achieve the health and fitness goals I have set.

21 Day Jumpstart Goals:

1. _____

2. _____

3. _____

6 Month Goals:

1. _____

2. _____

3. _____

12 Month Goals:

1. _____

2. _____

3. _____

I will do everything in my power to commit to the achievement
of the above set goals.

_____   _____
Signature   Date

JUMP-STARTING WEEK ONE EXERCISE

It's so easy for us in our ever-busy lives to create excuses for not exercising. I call these "exercuses." I haven't any extra time, I can't with my back pain, my blood pressure is too high, I get up so early as it is, my knees are shot, I'm too tired at night, it's too expensive to join that gym, I'm too old, blah, blah, blah...after 25 years of prescribing exercise sessions to individuals and groups of clients I have heard it all! So it's awesome that you have now committed to stopping that negative self talk and finished excusing yourself into inactivity! Not this time; now you are ready to initiate and complete this 21-day challenge!

Obviously you are ready for change because you have picked up this book and are ready to take one day at a time and start planting the seeds so you can reap the rewards! So congrats for going beyond making excuses and into making progress towards positive change!

At this point (or very soon) you should be geared up for your program; you may have bought the large exercise ball and strength training bands, maybe you bought new sneakers or exercise clothes, and you are gearing up mentally, ready to go for it!

Amongst my wellness peers, clients and staff, I am known to be a pretty challenging personal trainer. This is not just because I challenge my clients during their training sessions, but it's also because I expect a lot from people. I believe we all have great potential but we don't always expect enough of ourselves. Now is a good time to follow up with the written goals you have set. I encourage you to write out your plan as if you have already achieved your goals.

As you get mentally ready to tackle week one, here is **your Week One "Fit Tip"**—the law of expectation. The law of expectation says that what you deeply believe in, can mentally visualize, and expect to happen, you will achieve. This is very powerful. So *expect* to successfully complete the next 21-day program and expect to have great results!

Week one is a foundational week. Remember to start out nice and easy and alternate your cardio days with your strength days, drink your water and stretch after every workout! Good luck, and go for it!

Here is one of my favorite simple quotes. For you *Star Wars*™ fans, this quote is from Yoda when he was teaching Luke Skywalker to be a Jedi Master. Yoda said, *"Do or do not, there is no try."*

WEEK ONE EXERCISES

1. Ball Wall Squats
2. Push-ups
3. Lat Pulldowns (band)
4. Lunges
5. Standing Chest Press (band)
6. Seated Row (band)
7. Step-ups
8. Plank
9. Kneeling Cross Body
10. Ball Abdominal Curl

STRENGTH WORKOUT LOG

Week One

MONDAY		WEDNESDAY		FRIDAY	
Date:		**Date:**		**Date:**	
Warm-up for at least 10 minutes!		*Warm-up for at least 10 minutes!*		*Warm-up for at least 10 minutes!*	
Activity:		Activity:		Activity:	
Minutes:		Minutes:		Minutes:	
Heart Rate:		Heart Rate:		Heart Rate:	
Exercises	Reps	**Exercises**	Reps	**Exercises**	Reps
1. Ball Wall Squats		1. Ball Wall Squats		1. Ball Wall Squats	
2. Push-Ups		2. Push-Ups		2. Push-Ups	
3. Lat Pulldown*		3. Lat Pulldown*		3. Lat Pulldown*	
4. Lunges		4. Lunges		4. Lunges	
5. Standing Chest Press*		5. Standing Chest Press*		5. Standing Chest Press*	
6. Seated Row*		6. Seated Row*		6. Seated Row*	
7. Step-Ups		7. Step-Ups		7. Step-Ups	
8. Plank		8. Plank		8. Plank	
9. Kneeling Cross Body		9. Kneeling Cross Body		9. Kneeling Cross Body	
10. Ball Abdominal Curl		10. Ball Abdominal Curl		10. Ball Abdominal Curl	
STRETCH!		*STRETCH!*		*STRETCH!*	
Weight:		Weight:		Weight:	

These exercises require the use of an exercise band.

CARDIO WORKOUT LOG

Week One

TUESDAY	THURSDAY	SATURDAY
Date:	**Date:**	**Date:**
Activity:	Activity:	Activity:
Minutes:	Minutes:	Minutes:
Heart Rate:	Heart Rate:	Heart Rate:
Body Weight:	Body Weight:	Body Weight:
Comments:	**Comments:**	**Comments:**
**Remember to stretch at the end of each cardio session!	***Remember to stretch at the end of each cardio session!*	***Remember to stretch at the end of each cardio session!*

Balanced and Whole
Week One Food

WHAT ARE YOU EATING?

I ALWAYS START WITH THE good news: The first week you'll be concentrating on the "What" of your diet and not the "How Much." The bad news: The "What" will most likely be very different from your current diet so it will still be a big challenge!

The coolest thing about whole foods is that those that are the least calorically dense, that is, those containing the fewest calories, ounce for ounce, are also those that are the highest in vitamins, minerals, phytonutrients and fiber. Additionally, whole foods bring these nutrients in as a team; they work synergistically to provide optimal nutrition.

I'm talking about vegetables and fruits. When it comes to vegetables, many people don't eat enough, among other reasons, because they're short on time and we tend to focus on the "protein" when preparing meals. There is also less availability of fresh vegetables, in convenience form, than there is of just about everything else. There really is no excuse for not eating fruit; many of them, like oranges and bananas, come in single servings, individually WRAPPED portions-straight from Mother Nature!

The bottom line is that it isn't okay to just "skip" the foods we are eliminating for the 21-Day Jumpstart and not add in additional whole foods—namely vegetables! Even though non-starchy vegetables are lower in calories than much of what our staple diet will be, they are vital for providing the nutrients we require. They bring in vitamins, minerals, fiber and a host of phytonutrients with all the "super powers" you hear so much about in the media...as in, "Blueberries are good for your brain." Note to self: "Eat more blueberries."

If you focus on trying to eat all these "super foods" you can make yourself crazy, at least that's what my clients tell me. Here's what I tell them: If you eat an adequate variety of fruits and vegetables, in a variety of colors, and you let seasonality dictate which ones, in particular, you are focusing on in any given month, over the course of the year you will be getting all the nutrition you require. If you live in the northeast that means definitely overdose on berries and cherries in late spring and early summer when they are in season, local and less expensive. In mid to late summer, enter the amazing melons (watermelon, honeydew, cantaloupe, etc.), along with peaches and then plums. The fall brings us apples, pears, and cranberries, which carry us through to winter when the citrus peaks, shifting our focus to oranges and grapefruits. Citrus is an example of fruit that is seasonal but never locally grown for us Northeasterners.

Pomegranates in the fall are another example of these seasonal treats that are available and at their peak in the fall but never locally grown in the Northeast. Other fruits that are never locally grown but are available year-round include the tropical fruits—bananas, pineapples, and mangoes.

The rule: Favor locally grown whenever possible and rely on seasonal fruits at their peak during the non-growing seasons for your area. Supplement with the delicious fruits from outside your locale but don't make these your mainstay. Find out what produce is grown in your state, in each month, from a website by the National Resources Defense Council: www.simplesteps.org/eat-local

Also choose your vegetables by season. Consume a lot of dark, bitter leafy greens in the spring when they are harvested—they are naturally cleansing and detoxifying and will help you begin to shed a few of those extra pounds you may have accumulated over the winter.

In summer, you can get fresh organic corn, along with low-sugar fruits like zucchini, tomatoes, eggplants, and cucumbers; yes, even though they are on the Whole Foods list for vegetables, botanically they are fruits! In the fall eat cool-weather greens like kale, collards, broccoli and Brussels sprouts and "winter squash" like butternut, red kuri, delicata, acorn and spaghetti, to name a few!

These starchy winter squash will energize you along with root vegetables like sweet potatoes, turnips, rutabaga, celery root, onions, carrots, parsnips and beets. Root vegetables taste delicious in warming soups, stews, and casseroles or oven roasted with some aromatic herbs.

Spring again...time to eat the classic early spring bounty—peas, asparagus, radishes, artichokes and maybe try some you've never heard of like fiddleheads and fava beans!

When you let the season dictate your choices you are giving your body what it needs, when it needs it, and becoming more in tune with the environment in which you live. Produce grown locally and consumed soon after harvest has the highest nutrient content, as nutrients are lost through time and travel. Lastly, you are saving money eating this way and who doesn't love that?

This program is for people who don't necessarily want to know "why," but nevertheless, every ancient tradition strives to achieve harmony between the environment and the individual. This balance, which comes from the inside out, is a basic tenet of robust health. Even if you don't care why, knowing this little bit will nudge you toward letting nature assist you with your food choices.

When you are only "allowed" to eat whole foods, you suddenly realize the amazing variety of vegetables that are available. The best sources are the local farmer's markets, which may be year round if you live in California, but for many other areas, are limited to the growing seasons.

Natural markets typically offer locally grown organic produce and the larger stores offer fresh produce from all over the world. There's a whole wide spectrum of vegetables waiting to be discovered!

To learn more about farmer's markets in your area, you can consult the *Eat Well Guide*® which lists farmer's markets by zip code: www.eatwellguide.org

Another great resource to locate farms and farmer's markets near your home is www.localharvest.org.

If you grew up eating peas and carrots (the "square," frozen kind), you may have never developed your vegetable muscles. You'll be starting from scratch—tasting, trying and discovering many new ones. This is the fun part...discovering new foods that you enjoy eating and incorporating them into your diet forever. And that's success right there!

As you look over the "Whole Foods Lists" for fruits and vegetables at the end of this section, make your selections according to the season in which you are undertaking your 21-Day Jumpstart...color and variety are important, but remember that if you eat what is in season (preferably locally grown), you are getting the most vital, nutritious food available, and over the course of the year, you will have an ample variety of foods and the nutrients that come along with them.

What about the foods we're eliminating?

The Whole Foods lists are broken up by food group. The list for whole grains contains a long list of foods that are eliminated during the 21-Day Jumpstart. These foods include pasta, most breads, boxed rice and pasta "mixes," crackers, cookies, baked goods, waffles, flours and more. Is pasta a "bad" food that you should eliminate from your diet forever? For many of us the answer is no, meaning that including pasta in our diet, in moderation, is a healthy option.

Why eliminate pasta from the 21-Day Jumpstart?

Pasta is eliminated because it is not a whole food. Whole foods are in a form as close to their natural state as possible. Bread, pasta, and most of the foods on the eliminate list are made from grain that is pulverized (regardless of whether or not it is a "whole" grain). When we pulverize grain we break down the structure of the grain. In other words, even whole wheat flour, while retaining the vitamins and minerals that are naturally occurring in the wheat berry, is structurally changed by fine milling, which, in turn, changes the manner and speed by which it is broken down and digested in our bodies—thus it is no longer a "whole" food.

The speed at which carbohydrates are broken down in our bodies is measured by the glycemic index. Ironically, pasta (when not over-cooked) actually has a glycemic index similar to that of brown rice. Then why is brown rice included and pasta eliminated, you ask...

The simple answer is that brown rice is a whole food and pasta is not, but there are two other compelling reasons. Pasta contains gluten, a protein component of wheat, and many of us can benefit from reducing our consumption of it. Many processed foods contain wheat and many people suffer from overconsumption of wheat and gluten.

Although many 100% sprouted grain breads (which are permitted in the program) do contain gluten, it is generally a smaller amount and is much less problematic for many people than traditional wheat breads.[1]

Trigger Foods

The primary reason for eliminating pasta from our 21-day jumpstart is that pasta is a trigger food for many people.

A trigger food drives your hunger and compels you to keep eating. Cookies are an extreme and easy-to-understand example of a trigger food. I've always had this relationship with Thin Mints®—any Girl Scout cookie fans out there?

I can't eat just one Thin Mint without eating the whole sleeve; there-fore, Thin Mints® are a trigger food for me. These days I support the Girl Scouts by donating money to send cookies directly to our troops; and while I still enjoy eating them at parties and at friend's homes, I don't bring Thin Mints® into my house!

Pasta is a common and less obvious example. Many people don't feel satisfied after eating just one portion of pasta. We are more likely to keep eating the pasta than we are the brown rice. Perhaps it is be-cause in this country we are always served multiple portions of pasta and we have become conditioned to overeating it.

---

1 Note: The Balanced and Whole 21-Day Jumpstart Food Program is not a gluten-free diet.

Or maybe it's because pasta is a comfort food for many of us, or because whole foods like brown rice simply don't drive our "hunger" in the same way. Whatever the reason, once we're "off" these foods for a while, we crave them less.

Thus eliminating this hunger driver makes eating the appropriate portion size easier. Don't rely on being more disciplined; just remove the temptation!

This doesn't mean that we won't want to overeat pasta when it becomes available again. For many people the drive to overeat certain foods doesn't change; however, they may be able to successfully add these foods back into their diet by cooking only one portion size, always measuring portion sizes for certain foods like pasta, or only eating it once a week or on special occasions, as a "treat food."

Some people eat addictively or have very serious emotional eating issues. This program doesn't address those issues. Overeating is a continuum and many of us chronically overeat despite not having a food addiction or emotional eating issues that rise to the level of extreme food binging. Many of us are simply in the habit of eating more than we need to eat.

This is why the **Eating Habit Redesign for Week One** requires you to eat sitting down—your car doesn't count! This applies to everything you eat: meals, snacks, everything!

Sitting down sets the tone for a meal and forces us to slow down. Dr. John Douillard, an amazing Ayurvedic practitioner, author and teacher, taught me an ancient Ayurvedic saying that has helped me so much that I share it with all my clients. Roughly translated it means, "When you eat standing up, death is looking over your shoulder."[2]

If you remind yourself, every time you catch yourself eating standing up, that death is looking over your shoulder, you will be much more inclined to cop a squat!

Moms have a terrible habit of eating standing up and I was a chronic offender until I taught my children this axiom. Now, on the very rare

---

2   Used with permission from Dr. John Douillard, D.C., www.lifespa.com

occasion that my daughter spots me chewing while standing up, she just says, "There's someone looking over your shoulder, Mom!"

If you have children that are old enough to understand the larger concept here, I highly recommend sharing Dr. John Douillard's valuable teaching with them. You'll be teaching (and modeling) healthy eating habits, while encouraging yourself in making sitting down a habit. Children have memories like elephants and they love to catch us contradicting ourselves, so use that to your advantage. If you don't live alone, or even if you do, try enlisting others, wherever possible, to assist you in staying honest; becoming accountable to those around you will help you succeed!

Sitting down while you eat also prevents you from "picking" at food while you are preparing it, which can help you avoid mindlessly eating an extra half meal when cooking and preparing it. Additionally, if you have to attend any social functions, adhering to this Eating Habit Redesign will result in your eating less, guaranteed! Think about how competitive it can be to find a seat during cocktail hour at a catered event and even at many parties. How often are we standing up, chatting with someone, while munching on something?

Eliminating the television, phone, email and other distractions (while sitting down!) also forces you to focus on your food, and to be aware that it is mealtime. When your meal is over you will have a sense that you have been nourished. Likewise, when meal time is over, move on and stop thinking about food!

As we form new habits we establish for ourselves new patterns around food. We have the choice to continue to practice these new patterns or revert back to our old ones. Anyone who has ever gone home for the holidays can attest to how easily we fall back into old routines. We suddenly start eating foods that we no longer eat in our present life. It is very hard to resist these foods when we're in our childhood home because the habit is so ingrained and the environment, combined with the presence of the food, makes for powerful triggers.

Understanding how habits work helps us make better choices. If you're trying to change your eating habits, be wary of physical surroundings and emotional circumstances that trigger cravings for certain foods. Keeping a food diary helps you identify patterns in your eating. If you're replacing an afternoon snack break with an apple instead of a cup of coffee or a diet soda, try eating that apple in a different environment. Take a walk and find a new place to sit if you're used to eating or drinking at your desk.

The social fabric of your life is harder to change than your physical environment. You can't get rid of your family and friends and you may not be able to dictate what they eat (unless you're the mom!).

We can respect the choices of others and still make different choices for ourselves, as long as we aren't judgmental or condescending. I don't recommend trying to "convert" the people around you or implementing all the changes required for the 21-Day Jumpstart for your entire family as a "flash cut." If you live alone you can create your ideal home environment by purging all your processed foods; you can get the junk out, thus removing temptation.

The people you live with can sometimes provide added support. Try recruiting them to keep you accountable or enrolling them as a workout buddy—the more people on board the better! But don't try to force it on them; rather let them be inspired by the positive changes they see in you!

Your food diary will help you spot patterns in your eating, from what times you're most likely to crave/consume certain foods, to what foods, environments, people or circumstances are the biggest triggers for you. Is there something that makes you want to just sit on the couch and eat cheese?! We have to know what our food patterns are before we can change them...Week One is all about the What!

How will you feel?

Volumes have been written about sugar. Some say it is the most addictive drug we battle today. Since we are all starting our 21-Day Jumpstart in a different place, it's not possible to predict how each individual will feel in week one. If your current diet is high in added sugars, you may feel lousy for a couple of days.

Some people experience symptoms of headache, low energy, bad mood, etc. You may or may not experience this in week one, but if you do, be assured that the effects are temporary and that you will begin to feel better quickly ; most of my clients start to feel much better by Day Four.

What about alcohol?

Alcohol is a drug as well as a beverage. The same can be said for caffeine. This doesn't have to be controversial if you don't attach judgment to these substances.

The effects of these two beverages are very different... alcohol will impair your driving while caffeine will likely improve it; certainly when you're driving at night and feeling sleepy! If you are sensitive to caffeine, avoid having it in the late afternoon and evening when it can interfere with sleep.

Coffee, tea and alcohol are traditional foods with a long history of human consumption. I don't believe any of them needs to be eliminated from your 21-Day Jumpstart in the name of better health, but you may be well-served by objectively examining how much of them you are consuming and why.

There is no conclusive proof that any of these beverages, in moderation, causes health to decline, and current studies of all indicate moderate consumption has positive effects on health. If you have specific health conditions or circumstances for which alcohol or caffeine are contraindicated, you should not consume them.

Nor should you add any of these to your diet if it isn't already a part of it, just for purported "health benefits." Remember, there is no one perfect diet for everyone!

If you do enjoy alcohol, try to limit your alcohol consumption to one drink before a meal, preferably your main meal of the day. Alcohol works to "prime the pump" on your digestive system. If you have it right before a meal, the food you are eating will fulfill that hunger... this isn't true if you consume it apart from a meal, when it will likely result in your consuming additional calories and/or feeling the effects of the alcohol more acutely. This doesn't mean you have to chug your one glass of wine before dinner, instead, you can sip it with your dinner but limit it to one (5 ounce) glass. And, if you can save it as a weekend or more occasional treat, as opposed to including it every night, you'll be saving yourself some calories there.

While it's true that a larger man can metabolize more alcohol than a smaller woman, one of the goals of the 21-Day Jumpstart is to reduce weight. Keeping your alcohol consumption down to one glass of wine or beer or one mixed drink (without fruit juices or added sugars) before your meal will help you achieve your weight loss goals without giving up alcohol for the entire 21 days. Calories from alcohol are not a "free ride" and overconsumption of alcohol will sabotage your weight loss goals. Additionally, alcohol consumed before a meal is less likely to interfere with a good night's sleep. Alcohol can help you fall asleep but you may not sleep as soundly or for as long as you normally would when you consume alcohol very shortly before bedtime.

The timing for caffeine consumption is also important. If you have caffeine first thing in the morning or any other time on an empty stomach, it will interfere with natural hunger signals, as caffeine provides a short-term energy boost. One of the goals of the 21-Day Jumpstart is to help you tune into your body's natural signals and cues—merely changing the time at which you drink your coffee or tea can make a huge difference in how hungry you feel earlier in the day. Thus moving the time you consume your caffeine drink until after you've eaten helps you avoid playing "catch up" with food later in the day; it helps align your hunger with your body's energy needs.

Remember that week one doesn't require you to limit your food portion sizes except for dairy products!

You are required to add in certain foods and change the timing on others. These are enumerated in the section, Week One at a Glance.

At the end of this section, you will find Whole Foods Lists, including Foods to Eliminate, the Dairy Portion Chart, and sample meal and snack ideas. This information will be referenced throughout the program.

The sample meal ideas are broken down into 2 categories: Cookers and Builders. This is based on years of working with clients who, despite being successful in their health and weight loss goals, never cooked! It's best to cook your own food but if you are unable or unwilling, there are whole food options you can "build" in your own kitchen. When you eat foods prepared outside your home you're not in control of either the quantity or the quality of the ingredients used. And it can take longer to lose weight when you're getting most of your food from outside your home.

Your kitchen is your home's wellness center and it is my sincere hope that everyone feels motivated to prepare simple whole foods for their own meals. Just by taking advantage of frozen whole foods and learning some basic knife skills, you can expand your food repertoire and upgrade your nutrition. But, if you're just not into that, you can still learn how to healthily navigate the world of prepared food...i.e. how to make the best choices you can!

WEEK ONE AT A GLANCE

- **Water:** Make it the first thing into your body every morning! Fill a glass or canteen with water (8-12 oz.) and place it on your night table or other convenient location and consume it upon waking and at least 20 to 30 minutes before eating breakfast. This helps flush your organs and assists with elimination. Don't drink seltzer or other carbonated products. If you enjoy flavored water try soaking lemons, raspberries or other fruits or veggies in a pitcher of water overnight for added flavor.

- **Coffee or Tea:** Move your first cup to after breakfast. When consumed after food, it won't interfere with natural hunger signals. Some people find that coffee is a trigger for certain verboten foods...like donuts! If you discover it drives your cravings for sweets, you may be better off without the coffee. To avoid caffeine withdrawal headaches try having ½ cup of regular coffee mixed with decaf once a day in week one, 1/3 to ¼ cup in week 2 and then going entirely off it in week 3—caffeine withdrawal headaches are not necessary or helpful! If you love coffee, for a treat, try adding 1 tsp. maple syrup, 1 tsp. of unsweetened raw cocoa powder and a generous sprinkling of cinnamon into your coffee. Stir vigorously and enjoy!

- **Bread:** Consume only 100% sprouted grain bread. This may be tricky to find depending on where you live, but most natural food stores sell sprouted grain breads in the frozen section. *Food For Life®, Baking Company's Ezekiel 4:9®,* is 100% sprouted grain bread. Be sure to read labels carefully and only buy 100% sprouted grain bread, if possible. Many types of bread labeled "sprouted" are a combination of sprouted grain and conventional wheat flour.

- **Vegetables:** Eat a minimum of 2 servings a day. Add 2 servings of non-starchy vegetables a day to your diet. You are not limited to 2 servings a day; rather, 2 servings is the minimum. One serving= ½ cup of cooked vegetables (including cooked leafy greens) or raw "chunky" vegetables or 1 cup of raw leafy greens.

- **Extra Virgin Olive Oil:** Extra virgin olive oil is a great choice as your "go-to" added fat for vegetables, grains, salads and medium- to low-heat cooking (not frying). Be sure to buy extra virgin olive oil sold in a dark bottle or can as it is susceptible to damage by light.

- **Beans:** Add one tablespoon of cooked beans per day if you are not accustomed to eating beans. If you don't usually eat them, your body may need to get used to them slowly as beans can cause gas and discomfort in some people. Try adding a tablespoon to a salad or a grain dish. If you don't like beans or don't digest them well, try green beans, peas or edamame instead. Canned beans are convenient, but rinse and drain canned beans to eliminate extra salt.

- **Beverages:** Only beverages without any added sugars are allowed on the program. Eat whole fruits instead of consuming fruit juices. No artificially sweetened beverages are allowed (no "diet" drinks). If you have caffeine withdrawal from giving up diet soda, try a cup of freshly brewed, unsweetened black or green tea (iced or hot), or a cup of brewed coffee (or iced coffee). Flavored teas are also permitted.

Week One Daily Meal Skeleton

FIRST MORNING WATER

BREAKFAST

Whole Fruit

Choice of Food

+ 1 additional whole fruit daily

LUNCH/DINNER*

1 serving of vegetables

Animal protein (poultry, fish, meat, eggs, dairy),

with optional whole grain or starchy vegetable (never both) OR

Grain & Bean Combo OR

Starchy Vegetable & Bean Combo OR

Grain & Nuts or Seeds Combo OR

Starchy Vegetables & Nuts or Seeds Combo

* Lunch and Dinner have the same food choices/Choices are per meal

Eating Habit Redesign: Sit down when you eat.

WEEK ONE DAILY MEAL SKELETON GUIDELINES

- First Morning Water: Drink 8–12 ounces of water upon waking and at least 20 minutes before eating breakfast.

- "Choice of Food" for breakfast means you can eat any food you prefer. Try different foods and food combinations to discover which ones work best and keep you full the longest, i.e. allow you to go all the way to lunch without snacking.

- Food portion sizes are not limited, except dairy. Non-starchy vegetable portions are a minimum. One serving= ½ cup of cooked vegetables (including cooked leafy greens) or raw "chunky" vegetables or 1 cup of raw leafy greens.

- Food "Combos" listed are suggestions for satisfying meal options – no particular food combinations are required.

- Optional dairy = not more than 4 "wedges" per day. See Whole Foods Lists for Portion Sizes for dairy.

- Log all your daily foods and liquids (including water) on the food diary pages. When eating at home, measure serving sizes as best you can—use measuring cups for grains. This will help you in weeks 2 and 3.

- Eat within 15-45 minutes of vigorous exercise that is 1 hour in duration and higher intensity. If you will not be having a meal in the 15-45-minute window, eat a snack in that interval.

- Consume a minimum of 2 whole fruits per day. Use fruit as a dessert for lunch or dinner or have it alone as a snack.

- Snacks are chosen at your discretion. Always observe portion sizes for snacks. If you have a long period of time between meals (more than 4-6 hours), you will require snacks. If you are consuming 3 "square" meals, you don't need to snack if your energy is stable and you don't feel overly hungry.

Whole Foods Lists & Foods to Eliminate

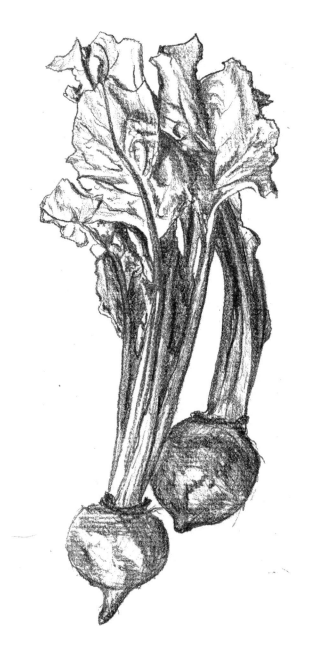

Fats & Oils

Unrefined Oils—The following list includes the unrefined oils commonly found in natural markets. There are many other unrefined oils like almond, pumpkin seed, avocado etc. Any unrefined oil, though many of them are very expensive, can be used to dress salads or vegetables.Some of them should not be heated. Only buy oils that are labeled as unrefined—many nut and seed oils found in the supermarket are refined and should be avoided.

Extra Virgin Olive Oil
(Unfiltered, Cold Pressed)
Unrefined Peanut Oil
Unrefined Sesame Oil
Unrefined Toasted Sesame Oil
(do not heat)

Unrefined Coconut Oil,
(Extra Virgin)
Red Palm Oil
Butter (Grass-Fed)
Ghee (Clarified Butter)

Refined oils—only for frying/high heat cooking. There are many other refined oils but these are very versatile.

Expeller Pressed Organic Canola[3]
Expeller Pressed Organic Safflower
Expeller Pressed Organic Sunflower

Note: Red Palm and Coconut oils are unrefined oils that can stand up to some higher heat cooking but there is a lot of variability by product, so follow manufacturer guidelines for temperature. These oils also impart their flavor to the food. Ghee (clarified butter), often used in Indian cooking, can also be used for higher heat cooking as ghee has a much higher smoke point than butter. Ghee is a dairy product so look for ghee that is organic.

---

3 Canola Oil is largely a genetically modified food. Canola oil labeled "USDA Organic" or "Non-GMO Project Verified" does not contain genetically modified organisms. For more information on non-gmo shopping visit http://www.nongmoshoppingguide. com or the Non-GMO Project at http://www.nongmoproject.org/

Basic Condiments

Shoyu (traditionally made, raw soy sauce)

Tamari (wheat-free soy sauce)

Ponzu

Hot sauces (Tabasco®, Cholula®, Sriracha, Harissa, etc.)

Vinegars (balsamic, apple cider, red wine, rice, umeboshi, champagne, sherry, etc.)

Gomasio (sea salt and sesame seed mixture)

Miso Paste

Mustard

Tomato Salsa (with no added sugar)

Prepared Pesto (with only extra virgin olive oil if you can find it)

Pesto Paste

Sun-dried Tomato Paste

Hot Chili Paste

Prepared Hummus (try for only extra virgin olive oil)

Eliminate: Ketchup, mayo and any sauces containing added sugar (barbeque sauces, etc.)

Spices: All spices are included, so use your favorites. If you don't do a lot of cooking here are a few basics:

cinnamon	cayenne pepper	thyme
chili powder	oregano	bay leaf
cumin	basil	red chili flakes
peppercorns	curry	granulated garlic

Note: I am a huge fan of Penzeys, including many of their spice blends that make getting more flavor simpler. Penzeys spices are available at their stores or on the web at www.Penzeys.com

Sweeteners

Raw Honey

Real Maple Syrup

Fruit

Apple	Grape	Orange
Apricot	Grapefruit	Papaya
Banana	Honeydew	Peach
Bilberry	Huckleberry	Pear
Blackberry	Jackfruit	Pineapple
Blueberry	Jambul	Plum
Cantaloupe	Kiwi	Pomegranate
Cherry	Kumquat	Prune
Clementine	Lemon	Raisin
Cranberry	Lime	Rambutan
Currant	Lychee	Raspberry
Date	Mango	Strawberry
Fig	Mangostein	Tangerine
Gooseberry	Nectarine	Watermelon

Legumes & Beans

Note: Immature legumes are young legumes we eat from the garden; examples are edamame (young soy beans), green beans and peas. These are listed under vegetables but are truly legumes. The mature and dried varieties are on the list below.

Aduki	Lentil
Black (black turtle)	Lima
Navy	Mung Peas
Cannellini	Mung Beans
Chickpeas (garbanzo)	Pinto
Fava (fresh or dried)	Red Beans
Great Northern	Soy Beans
Green and Yellow Peas (dried)	White Kidney
Kidney	

Peanuts are legumes and whole peanuts or natural peanut butter (no added sugars or hydrogenated oils) are permitted. The portion size for peanuts is same as other nuts—1 ounce—unlike the rest of the legumes!

All other nuts and seeds, and nut and seed butters that don't contain added sugars or added oils, are also permitted in the 21-Day Jumpstart. There is no Whole Foods List for nuts but there is a Nut Chart in the Appendix C on page 170, which provides the approximate number of nuts in a one-ounce serving.

Eliminate:
Canned Vegetarian Chili with added sugars (many contain
    evaporated cane juice...aka sugar!)
Canned Baked Beans with added sugars (make your own!)
Canned Bean soups with added sugars

Animal Foods & Seafood

All species of unprocessed animal foods or seafood are included. Strive to buy organic, naturally raised (grass-fed/pasture-raised/free-range) for meats, poultry and eggs, and wild caught for seafood, if possible.

Eliminate all processed meats and seafood:
    Bacon
    Canned or bottled chili or other canned meats
    "Chicken nuggets" or other processed chicken—any prepared
        chicken with "coating"
    Deli meats (cold cuts)
    Fish sticks or other processed seafood items
    Jerky, fried or smoked meats or fish
    Meat pies or "Pot Pies"—frozen or fresh
    Commercially prepared quiches
    Prepared salads (tuna, egg, chicken)
    Sausages
    Hot Dogs

Dairy & Eggs

Strive to buy organic and free-range eggs and organic grass-fed dairy, if possible. All species of dairy are included—cow, goat, sheep, etc.

   Eggs
   Whole milk
   Buttermilk
   Unsweetened Almond Milk
   Unsweetened Soy Milk
   Whole, plain yogurt
   Whole, plain Kefir
   Sour Cream
   Cottage Cheese
   Ricotta Cheese
   Other cheeses (hard and soft), (raw milk if possible)

Eliminate all dairy products and non-dairy substitutes to which sugar or artificial sweeteners are added:

   Flavored yogurt (sugar or artificial sweetener, including
      non-dairy)
   Flavored milks (including non-dairy, if sweetened)
   Processed cheese foods (including non-dairy)
   Puddings (including non-dairy)

Portion Sizes for Dairy

Portion sizes are limited for dairy products. I recommend, if you consume dairy, you consume full-fat dairy and have smaller daily portions. Full-fat dairy products are whole foods and the fat aids in the absorption of fat soluble vitamins present in dairy foods. The fat also mitigates the impact that the simple sugars present in dairy have on your blood sugar.

   For the entire 21-Day Jumpstart, use the dairy portions given in "wedges" to eat any combination amounting to no more than 4 wedges daily.

If you don't normally consume any dairy do not start eating it for the 21-Day Jumpstart unless you like it, are able to digest it well and wish to eat it. Dairy is an optional food.

If you are not consuming dairy be sure to eat dark leafy greens, broccoli and nuts and seeds like almonds and sesame seeds to provide your body with calcium.

Note: Non-dairy milks, like almond and soy, are not whole foods. They are included, for convenience, for people who do not consume dairy milk. It is important to consume only the unsweetened varieties. Soy is predominantly a genetically modified crop. If you wish to avoid GMO's, purchase soy products that are labeled "USDA Organic" or "Non-GMO Project Verified".

Coconut milk is often used in Thai cooking and adds richness to soups and stews. The coconut milk below does not refer to the non-dairy refrigerated beverage.

Dairy Portion Sizes

1 Wedge	2 Wedges	3 Wedges
1 tbsp. cream cheese	4 oz.(½ cup) cottage cheese	8 oz. plain, whole milk yogurt (any species)
1 tbsp. feta or other crumbled or shredded cheese	2 tbsp. crumbled or shredded cheese (hard or soft)	8 oz. whole milk
2 tbsp. grated Parmesan cheese	cheese stick (1 oz.)	8 oz. whole milk kefir
2 tbsp. sour cream	¼ cup whole milk ricotta cheese	8 oz. buttermilk
8 oz. unsweetened almond milk	8 oz. unsweetened soy milk	2 oz. (¼ cup) coconut milk

Vegetables

Artichoke
Avocado
Asparagus
Broccoli
Broccoli Rabe
Beet
Brussels Sprout
Bok Choy
Bell Pepper
Burdock Root
Butternut Squash
Cauliflower
Cabbage
Carrot
Celery
Cilantro
Chives
Collard Greens
Corn
Cucumber
Chili Pepper
Celeriac (celery
   root)
Cassava (yuca)
Chicory
Dandelion
Daikon Radish
Dulse (sea
   vegetable)
Eggplant

Endive
Escarole
Fiddlehead Ferns
Fennel
Garlic
Ginger
Green Beans
Hearts of Palm
Hijiki (sea
   vegetable)
Horseradish
Jalapeno Pepper
Jerusalem
   Artichoke
Jicama
Kale
Kohlrabi
Kombu (sea
   vegetable)
Leek
Lettuce (all types)
Mache
Mizuna
Mushroom (all
   types)
Mustard greens
Onions
Okra
Olives
Parsley

Parsnip
Peas (green, snow
   and snap)
Potato
Pumpkin
Purslane
Radicchio
Radish
Rhubarb
Rutabaga
Spinach
Squash (all)
Shallot
Scallions
Sorrel
Sprouts
Sweet Potato
Swiss Chard
Tomato
Tomatillo
Turnip
Taro
Tatsoi
Wakame (sea
   vegetable)
Watercress
Water Chestnut
Yam
Zucchini

Live cultured vegetables such as pickles, sauerkraut, and kimchi are allowed (and encouraged!) on the program. Naturally fermented foods contain probiotics which help us maintain a healthy gut flora. As fermented foods have become more popular, the variety of live cultured vegetables has increased. In addition to cabbage, an old standby, you can also find live cultured beets, daikon radish and carrots!

A little goes a long way with fermented vegetables – try adding a great tasting pickle to your brown bag lunch and/or having a tablespoon or two of kimchi (available in differing levels of spiciness) or other live cultured vegetables as part of your lunch or dinner meal.

Whole Grains

All unprocessed whole grains are permitted. This is not a complete list but includes many whole grains options.

    Brown Rice
    Basmati Rice* (including white basmati)
    Buckwheat (kasha)
    Farro
    Oats (steel cut and old fashioned)
    Quinoa
    Barley
    Bulgur (cracked wheat)
    Millet
    Kamut
    Rye berries
    Spelt
    Wheat berries

*Basmati rice, including white basmati, has a lower glycemic index than other types of rice. Additionally, there is ongoing research pertaining to the presence of inorganic arsenic (the most toxic form of arsenic) in rice, levels of which are much higher in **all types** of brown rice.

White basmati rice, grown in California, India or Pakistan, and sushi rice grown in the U.S., have much lower levels of inorganic arsenic than other rice, according to a November 2012 analysis by Consumer Reports. Although brown basmati has significantly less inorganic arsenic than other types of brown rice, it is still much higher in inorganic arsenic than white basmati.[4]

This underscores the importance of eating a variety of foods, including a variety of whole grains.

---

[4] Copyright 2012 by Consumers Union of U.S., Inc. Yonkers, NY 10703-1057, d/b/a/ Consumer Reports, a nonprofit organization and publisher of the Consumer Reports family of products. Reprinted with permission from the November 2012 issue of Consumer Reports for educational purposes only. No commercial use or reproduction permitted. www.ConsumerReports.org.

Grains to Eliminate
    Bread (eat only 100% sprouted grain bread)
    Flours (including grits,* cornmeal and polenta)
    Pasta (all types)
    Pizza
    Bagels
    Muffins
    Granola** (commercially prepared)
    Crackers or flatbreads
    Boxed rice and pasta mixes
    Boxed breakfast cereals
    Tortilla chips and other corn chips
    Pretzels and all other packaged snack foods
    Baked goods, such as cake, cookies, etc.
    Pancakes
    Waffles
    Frozen burritos and other breakfast products
    Energy bars or other packaged food bars

*Grits, cornmeal and polenta are 100% whole grain corn but they are basically corn "flours" and the 21-Day Jumpstart eliminates most flour products. This doesn't mean they are not part of a healthy whole foods diet for the long haul.

**If you can't survive without some granola in your yogurt or oatmeal, look for organic granola with no more than 4 to 5 grams of sugar, per serving, or try making your own! Many packaged granolas are high in added sugars and refined oils. Use 2 tbsp. as your portion size.

➤ *Consult the recipe section, in Appendix C on page 171, for information on cooking rice and other grains.*

Rules for selecting Sample Meals

1. Use the food diary pages provided to log your food. It is important to see what, how much and how often you are eating, including the times you eat meals and any snacks.

2. Eat enough breakfast to get you through until lunch without a snack. Hint: If you're hungry enough to eat your shoes two hours after breakfast you either didn't eat enough food or didn't eat the right combination of food. If you notice that you get hungry very quickly after eating a carbohydrate-based breakfast (like grain and vegetables), you may do better eating more protein or fat in the morning. Try a few different types of breakfasts and see which ones work best for you. Adding nuts or other fats to a grain-based breakfast may also keep you full longer.

3. Don't choose the same "entrée" more than once per day. For example, if you eat eggs for breakfast, don't eat eggs for lunch or dinner. Likewise for avocadoes, peanut butter, ricotta cheese, etc. Any food you choose as the "main course" for a meal should not be repeated in the same day. For dairy foods, cross off the dairy wedges on your daily food diary as you use them, to easily track servings. As the weeks progress, keep daily portion restrictions in mind when selecting sample meals (pay special attention to nuts, nut butters, added fats and dairy foods) and do not exceed the suggested daily limits.

4. Limit bread to one meal per day; if you're eating a sandwich for breakfast, choose lunch and dinner options that don't include bread.

5. Avoid all commercial salad dressings when possible. For salads you purchase outside your home, use extra virgin olive oil (1 or 2 tsp.) and vinegar as a dressing, if available, or else order dressing on the side and use two tablespoons. If you are making salad at home, try umeboshi vinegar, a very tart and salty Asian vinegar that will liven up your greens, or a good quality apple cider vinegar as a change from balsamic and red wine vinegars.

6. Practice moderation with your use of salty condiments and any canned or prepared foods like salsa, sauces, hummus, olives or grape leaves. To "balance out" your daily salt intake, be mindful of the types of condiments you are using in a single day. If you use soy sauce, for example, in one meal, don't choose a sample recipe or make a recipe of your own that includes a salty condiment for another meal in the same day. Foods with a "% Daily Value" for Sodium of 20 or more, per serving, are salty.

7. Feel free to swap out any of the meals.

8. A list of snack ideas is provided. Fresh fruit is great between meals, if the interval is short. For longer intervals, you may also need some fat or protein like a tablespoon of nut butter, or an ounce of olives. Stay within the daily portion guidelines for dairy if it is a part of your snack.

9. Meal Repetition: Avoid eating the same thing every day! Nutrient intake increases with variety. Eating the same foods repeatedly also exposes you to a larger quantity of any undesirable substances present in those foods. Inorganic arsenic in rice is one such example. Eating raw oats, which are higher in phytates than cooked oats, as in the *Grab & Go Overnight Oats* recipe is another. Eating these foods less frequently makes life simpler!

Sample Meal Ideas

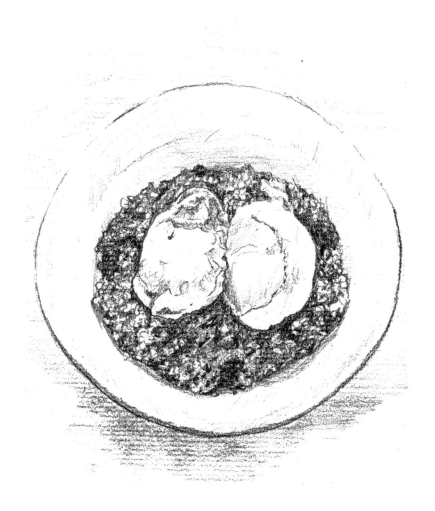

SAMPLE BREAKFAST MEALS — Cookers

1. **Breakfast Porridge:** Steel cut oats or other grain porridge with an optional tablespoon or two of nuts or seeds. Re-heat cooked grains with water, milk, or non-dairy milk and add a sprinkle of cinnamon, a ½ tsp. of vanilla and/or one teaspoon of maple syrup or raw honey.

    Alternatively, add fresh fruit such as ½ cup blueberries.

2. **Poached Eggs*/3 Ways:** Poach two eggs and plop on a scoop of leftover grain. For some zing, sprinkle eggs with a hot sauce like Tabasco®, Chulula® or Sriracha.

    Alternatively, sauté baby greens like spinach or arugula (use ½ of a 5 oz. clamshell package or about 3 cups) in 1 tbsp. of extra virgin olive oil, sprinkle with pinch of sea salt, and drop poached eggs on top of greens.

    Super basic 3rd option: Poach two eggs and plop on toasted, sprouted grain bread—top eggs with hot sauce or try chopped fresh chives, they're awesome...wipe up the yolk with your bread corners!

3. **Breakfast Sauté:** Sauté vegetables of choice (onion, pepper, etc.) in 1 tbsp. extra virgin olive oil and add diced leftover poultry or meat (½-1 cup), until heated through. Add 2 handfuls of baby spinach and sauté another minute or two until spinach wilts. Season to taste.

4. **Veggie Sauté:** Sauté fresh vegetables (as above) and add a scoop of leftover grain (½–1 cup) to sauté to heat through when veggies are cooked.

5. **Avocado Power:** Slice avocado (½ Hass-type avocado or ¼ of the larger type) over salad greens, sprinkle with sea salt and balsamic vinegar, or eat an "open-face" sandwich by slicing

See recipe section, Appendix C, page 178

avocado and placing on toasted sprouted whole grain bread, sprinkling with sea salt and drizzling with balsamic vinegar.

6. **Salmon Power:** Open and spread a salmon pouch (3.5 oz.) over salad greens. Drizzle with balsamic vinegar or eat salmon "open face" on top of a slice of toasted, sprouted whole grain bread spread with a thin layer of cream cheese (1 tbsp.). Optionally, top salmon with sliced red onion or other veggie, if desired.

7. **Breakfast Bean Skillet:** Sauté ½ of medium onion (about ½ cup chopped onion) in 1 tbsp. extra virgin olive oil for about 5 minutes until softened (sprinkle with pinch of sea salt). Add ½ cup of black beans (or substitute ½ cup of pinto beans) and ¼ cup of salsa and cook a minute or two more, until heated through. Sprinkle with two tablespoons of shredded cheddar cheese and ¼ of an avocado, diced small, if using the smaller Hass-type avocado—if using larger avocado, use ¼ cup diced.

    Optional "Turbo Boost"—If you just worked out and want to add a little more oomph to this breakfast option, poach one egg and plop on top of your Bean Skillet bowl; the yolk will create a scrumptious "icing" for your beans.

SAMPLE BREAKFAST MEALS — Builders

1. **Grab & Go Overnight Oats*** (no cooking required) or prepare frozen steel cut oats according to package directions and eat with a tablespoon or two of nuts or seeds, dash of cinnamon and 1 tsp. real maple syrup and/or fresh fruit. Purchase frozen, prepared steel cut oats with no added sugars.

2. **Cheesy Toast:** "Open-face" toasted, sprouted whole grain bread with ¼ cup ricotta cheese sprinkled with sea salt and chopped, fresh chives or other seasonal veggies (sliced tomatoes, red onion, etc.).

3. **The Nutty Banana:** "Open-face" toasted, sprouted grain bread with 2 tbsp. of peanut or almond butter and a banana, sliced long-ways. Optional: Top with another slice of toast for full sandwich.

4. **Portable Eats:** Cheese stick and an apple (or other fruit) or one ounce of nuts** and fruit.

5. **Eggs and Toast:** Two hard-boiled eggs with slice of buttered, sprouted whole grain toast. Optional: Slice hard-boiled egg and place on top of plain toast—sprinkle with hot sauce, if desired, but be careful...hard-boiled eggs fall off!

6. **Breakfast Salad:** Salad with ½ cup cottage cheese or with ½ cup of beans and/or hard-boiled egg(s). Another Option: ½ cup cottage cheese with fruit.

7. **Yogurt Parfait:** Plain yogurt with one or two tbsp. nuts or seeds, or granola and cut fresh fruit.

*See recipe section, Appendix C, page 179

**See nut chart in Appendix C, page 170

SAMPLE LUNCH MEALS — Cookers

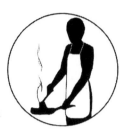

1. **"Dinner Take Two":** Dinner leftovers make the best lunch! Lean animal foods (chicken, seafood or meat) with optional leftover grain or starchy vegetable or vegetarian combo with cooked or raw vegetables and/or side salad.

2. **Julie's Chicken Fried Rice*** and side salad.

3. **Yam Salad:** 1 to 1 ½ cups of roasted sweet potato wedges* over 2–3 cups salad greens with ½ oz. of nuts** (pecans are delicious). Use ¼ cup of tahini sauce* instead of conventional salad dressing.

4. **Homemade Chili or Hearty Bean Soup,** (serving size about 1 cup for chili, 2 cups for soup, as main course) with optional ½ cup of cooked grain and side salad or cucumber wheels.

5. **Stuffed Potato:** Mound 1 cup homemade chili on a small whole, split baked potato(sweet or white) or larger baked potato half (skin on), top with 1 tablespoon of grated cheddar cheese and 1 tablespoon of sour cream and fresh chives or chopped scallions, with side of steamed broccoli.

6. **Mediterranean Spaghetti Squash,*** and side salad with 1-2 hard-boiled eggs.

7. **Farro Salad*** with Italian-Style Green Beans.*

*See recipe section, Appendix C, page 180

**See nut chart in Appendix C, page 170

SAMPLE LUNCH MEALS — Builders

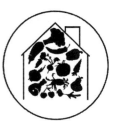

1. **Avocado Sandwich**: "Open-face," ½ avocado, sliced, with one slice of Swiss cheese (try Emmentaler!) and 1 cup of greens (arugula is delicious!) on top of toasted, sprouted, whole grain bread, spread with mustard. Raw veggies on side.
2. **Pesto Tomato Bowl*** with side of cucumber sticks.
3. **Tuna White Bean Salad,*** optional toast triangles (toasted slice of sprouted whole grain bread diagonally cut into 4 triangles) and carrot sticks on side.
4. **Tapas**: Cheese stick with apple or pear slices, ¼ cup of hummus with carrot sticks for dipping and 3 to 5 grape leaves (*Mediterranean Organic*™ brand is delicious!)
5. **Chicken Lettuce Wraps*** **with Peanut Sauce,*** side of carrot sticks.
6. **Hummus sandwich**: Toast sprouted, whole grain bread and spread ¼ cup of hummus on top. Sprinkle hummus with ½ tbsp. toasted sesame seeds (see page 180). Cut 4 cucumber slices thinly and nestle into hummus. Peel a large carrot and use potato peeler to grate clean carrot on top of cucumber slices. Eat "open face" or top with an additional slice of toast.
7. **Chopped Salad**: Chop 2–3 cups romaine, one hard-boiled egg, ½ cup cucumber slices, ½ of jalapeno pepper, seeds removed, and 5 Kalamata olives. Add ½ cup of cannellini beans and two tablespoons sliced almonds to chopped veggies. Toss with two tbsp. of your favorite vinaigrette.

*See recipe section, Appendix C, page 186

SAMPLE DINNER MEALS — Cookers

1. **Baked Cod, Italian Style*** with green salad.
2. **Chicken or Shrimp Stir Fry** over grain with side salad. Cut boneless, skinless chicken breast into narrow strips and sauté in wok or skillet until browned on both sides (about 5 minutes). Add your favorite raw vegetables, such as broccoli, snow peas, and diced yellow onion, etc. and seasonings such as 1 teaspoon of grated fresh ginger and a pinch of sea salt or 1 to 2 teaspoons tamari or shoyu sauce and ¼ cup of water; continue cooking until vegetables are tender—about 5-10 minutes. Sprinkle with one tablespoon toasted sesame seeds and enjoy over basmati rice or whole grain of your choice.

   If using cooked shrimp, add shrimp to skillet after vegetables are cooked to heat through and season.

   If using raw shrimp, larger ones may need to be cut. Add raw shrimp at the same time you add your vegetables.
3. **Roasted Pork Tenderloin with Onion & Apples,*** grain pilaf and spinach salad.
4. **Turkey Meatloaf,*** roasted asparagus* and green salad.
5. **Black Bean Patties***, pickle slices and green salad.
6. **Skirt Steak with Chimichurri,*** green bean and arugula salad.*
7. **Greek Quinoa Salad,*** roasted sugar snap peas. Rinse and stem sugar snap peas. Coat baking dish with tsp. organic canola oil (use brush or paper towel) and roast in 375 degree oven for 10 minutes. After baking, toss peas with 1 tbsp. extra virgin olive oil and sprinkle with sea salt.

*See recipe section, Appendix C, page 189

SAMPLE DINNER MEALS — Builders

1. **Easy Brown Rice & Beans,*** or **Easy Brown Rice & Peas*** and large green salad.

2. **Grilled Chicken or Shrimp over Spinach Salad:** Purchase prepared grilled chicken breast or cooked shrimp. Slice and arrange over a spinach salad. Add sliced red onion, thinly sliced radish, 1 or 2 tablespoons of goat cheese and a tablespoon or two of sliced almonds. Dress with 2 tablespoons of dressing of your choice or 1-2 tsp. extra virgin olive oil and as much vinegar as desired.

3. **Pesto Rice Salad with Edamame & Walnuts,*** side of carrot sticks and yogurt sauce* for dipping.

4. **Rotisserie chicken,** "stir fry" frozen mixed vegetables and arugula salad.

5. **Super Salmon Salad*** over baby greens or stuffed into hollowed-out tomato or pepper with side salad.

6. **Prepared Grilled Fish Salad:** Purchase prepared grilled or broiled fish fillet, cut up and set aside. Thinly slice red onion, tomato, and cucumber. Add one tablespoon of sliced almonds to sliced veggies and toss with mixed greens (including thinly sliced raw lacinato kale, if desired) and 2 tbsp. Balsamic Vinaigrette.* Top tossed salad with cut-up fish fillet and sprinkle with one teaspoon capers.

7. **Green Chicken Salad*** over arugula or baby greens, or, if you're a cooker, nestle your chicken salad in a roasted delicata squash "boat" (half of an oven-roasted delicata squash, skin on).

*See recipe section, Appendix C, page 195

SAMPLE MEALS FOR EATING OUT

1. **Deli/Café/Sandwich Shop**: Salad with lean meat or seafood or cup of lentil or other bean soup with optional scoop of rice and side salad. If ½ and ½ options are available, choose soup and salad.

2. **Mexican**: Opt for a "naked" burrito (no tortilla shell). Request either a ½ portion of brown rice, black or pinto beans, vegetables, tomato salsa, and lettuce or, if ordering meat or chicken, skip the rice and just add beans and veggies. Ask for sour cream and/or cheese on side and portion it. **Skip:** Guacamole and Queso sauce.

3. **Asian**: Brown rice and sautéed vegetables with minimal sauce (i.e. sautéed string beans with garlic, sautéed eggplant, etc.), cup of broth-based soup (hot and sour/Tom Yum), and/or lean meat or seafood, vegetables and brown rice. **Skip:** Fried noodles, noodles, Pad Thai, wontons, fried rice, scallion pancakes, shrimp toast, egg and spring rolls, fried or tempura-style meats or seafood, fish or shrimp cakes and fortune cookies—many contain trans fats! You can still read your fortune!!

4. **Diner**: Salad with chicken, hard-boiled eggs or avocado. Side of cooked veggies. Side of grape leaves. Lean meat or seafood with vegetables and side salad. "Naked" veggie burger with side salad. **Skip:** Home fries and toast, French or sweet potato fries, tuna or egg salads, Greek salad with a copious amount of feta cheese and all fried foods (falafel, etc.).

5. **Restaurant**: Broiled, wild-caught seafood or other lean animal food with side salad and vegetables. Vegetarian entrées are fine but be wary of those containing cheese, dairy-based sauces or puff pastry. **Skip:** Rolls and bread, mashed white potatoes, etc.

6. **Italian:** Traditional Italian restaurants may offer beans and greens like escarole and beans. Alternatively, order a bowl of minestrone with a side salad and a side of cooked greens—try broccoli rabe, escarole or sautéed spinach. Broiled seafood over a bed of greens is also a great choice. **Skip:** Pasta, pizza, bread, and breaded or fried vegetables, meat or seafood—almost everything!

7. **Sushi:** One roll (typically 6-8 pieces). Opt for cooked or raw seafood or vegetarian rolls. Add a cup of Miso soup and/or side salad. **Skip:** Tempura-style or fried seafood or meat.

8. **Korean:** Bibimbap is a bowl of sticky rice topped with vegetables, sometimes meat or seafood and a poached or fried egg. My favorite way to eat it is just the rice and vegetables topped with a poached egg, as it is a simple, whole foods entrée.

9. **Indian:** Choose light vegetable curries, dal, Chana Masala, Chicken Tikka Masala, Tandoori Chicken, Saag or Palak Paneer, etc. **Skip:** Samosas and other deep-fried foods, heavy curries and dishes with a lot of cream and butter.

10. **Greek:** Choose broiled seafood over a bed of greens and ask for cucumber slices, instead of pita, for dipping in hummus and babaganoush. **Skip:** Spanakopita and falafel and mind the quantity of feta in your salad!

11. **Fast Food:** Many of the fast food chains offer salad options. Avoid ordering salads topped with breaded or fried animal foods. Use ½ package of the dressing.

Snack Ideas

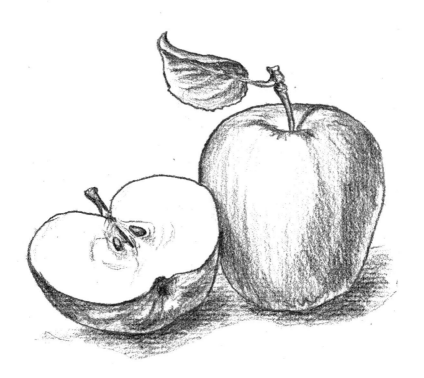

SNACK CHART

CRISPY	SWEET
• Apple: Eat whole or dip slices in 1 tbsp. nut butter or 1/4 cup of hummus • Veggie Sticks: dip in ¼ cup hummus, bean dip or yogurt sauce (recipe page 202). • Nuts: (½ - 1 oz) See nut chart page 170 • Sunflower or Pumpkin seeds: (¼ cup) • Baked Chickpeas: (¼ - ½ cup) recipe page 205 • Kale Chips: or other roasted vegetable "chips" (½ - 1 cup) recipe page 204	• Pineapple Chunk Skewer or strawberries or other sweet cut fruits. (1 cup) • Roasted Sweet Potato Wedges: (½ cup – about 10 wedges) recipe page 181 • Rice pudding: (½ cup) recipe page 206 • Prunes (4) • Frozen Grapes (1 cup): Put single serving portion of grapes in sandwich baggie and freeze. • Stuffed Banana: Leave peel on banana and slit long ways through peel. Stuff with 1 tbsp. nut butter and drizzle with 1 tsp. raw honey. Cover in foil and bake for 10–15 minutes at 350°F to melt and soften. Scoop with spoon.
SAVORY	SMOOTH
• Olives: (5 or 6) • Pickle • Edamame: (1 cup), soybeans in pod, dipped in sea salt (discard pods). • Stuffed Radishes: (6) Cut a deep trench when removing stem of clean radishes. Divide ½ tbsp. butter into 6 rectangles and press butter into trench. Sprinkle with sea salt. • Raw Milk Parmesan Cheese: (1 inch cube) • Oven Roasted Brussels Sprouts: (1 cup) recipe page 203	• Plain Yogurt with fruit: ½ cup yogurt with cut fruit • Cheese Stick • Avocado Slices: (¼ of a Hass-type avocado or ¼ cup) drizzle with balsamic vinegar and/or olive oil and sprinkle of sea salt • "Green Mousse": Blend ¼ cup of avocado, ½ banana and ¼ cup of water in Vitamix® or blender until smooth. Eat with spoon. • Cottage Cheese: ½ cup (4 oz.) with optional cut fruit • Unsweetened Applesauce: ½ cup (try making your own!)

Note: Nut Chart and all recipes can be found in Appendix C

Week One Food Diary

Date_____

First AM Water

Dairy

TIME	AMOUNT	FOOD/BEVERAGE	SAT DOWN? Y/N	HUNGER RATING (0-5)

What went well? _____

Struggles? _____

What to do differently tomorrow? _____

Week One Food Diary

Date_____

First AM Water

Dairy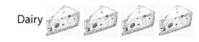

TIME	AMOUNT	FOOD/BEVERAGE	SAT DOWN? Y/N	HUNGER RATING (0-5)

What went well? _____

Struggles? _____

What to do differently tomorrow? _____

Week One Food Diary

Date_____

First AM Water 🥛   Dairy 🧀 🧀 🧀 🧀

TIME	AMOUNT	FOOD/BEVERAGE	SAT DOWN? Y/N	HUNGER RATING (0-5)

What went well? _____

Struggles? _____

What to do differently tomorrow? _____

Week One Food Diary

Date_____

First AM Water

Dairy

TIME	AMOUNT	FOOD/BEVERAGE	SAT DOWN? Y/N	HUNGER RATING (0-5)

What went well? _____

Struggles? _____

What to do differently tomorrow? _____

Week One Food Diary

Date_____

First AM Water 🥛

Dairy

TIME	AMOUNT	FOOD/BEVERAGE	SAT DOWN? Y/N	HUNGER RATING (0-5)

What went well? _____

Struggles? _____

What to do differently tomorrow? _____

Week One Food Diary

Date_____

First AM Water 　　　　　　　　　Dairy

TIME	AMOUNT	FOOD/BEVERAGE	SAT DOWN? Y/N	HUNGER RATING (0-5)

What went well? _____

Struggles? _____

What to do differently tomorrow? _____

Week One Food Diary

Date_____

First AM Water   Dairy

TIME	AMOUNT	FOOD/BEVERAGE	SAT DOWN? Y/N	HUNGER RATING (0-5)

What went well? _____

Struggles? _____

What to do differently tomorrow? _____

21-Day Jumpstart Food and Exercise Journal
Week One

____ / ____ / ____ — ____ / ____ / ____

Please log your feelings, thoughts, and comments on how your daily nutrition and exercise has been going during this first week.

_____

_____

_____

_____

_____

_____

_____

_____

_____

_____

_____

_____

_____

_____

_____

_____

_____

_____

_____

_____

_____

Balanced and Whole
Week Two Exercise

WEEK ONE EXERCISE ADAPTATIONS

YOU MADE IT THROUGH WEEK one—you are doing great! Now that you are stimulating your body with new strength training and cardiovascular exercise, several physiological adaptations have started almost immediately. These changes occur throughout the body, but the most significant modifications include improvements to your muscles, bones and cardiovascular system. Your muscles start a process called hypertrophy, which is changes in the size of your muscle fibers and an increase in the number of muscle contractile proteins. These adaptations are the initial phase of your body's boosting its metabolism and enhancing its ability to burn fat.

Like the muscles, your bones are also responding to the new exercise stimulus. Your bones are stressed during exercise and by adding this impact, the tendons and muscles are pulling on the bones. This added "strain" to the bones stimulates the bones to become more dense.

Your cardiovascular system is going through many adaptations as well as a result of the aerobic exercise you are doing. Your heart starts to become more efficient at pumping and delivering fresh blood to the working muscles. Improved blood volume increases blood capillary density and function to deliver more blood to the trained muscles improving your ability to perform intense exercise. As a result, your resting heart rate and blood pressure levels decrease.

As you go through these beginning stages of transformation, your body is still adjusting to the work load. You still may be a little sore from the new muscle stimulus. At this point it is crucial to remain consistent and not skip any days of exercise except for your one rest day per week.

JUMP-STARTING WEEK TWO EXERCISE

"Repetition is the mother of skill," it has been said. If you continue to do the same things over and over and repeat familiar motor skills, the body memorizes this action on a neuromuscular level—this is called "muscle memory." As you continue to stimulate the body again and again, it becomes automatic or second nature, cognitively and physically. Exercises are now becoming easier to perform without as much conscious effort. Your body is beginning to ask for that movement. After your rest day, your body will be telling you it's time to get up and walk. And when you have given your body the ample 48 hours of rest between your strength workouts, your body will be looking for more muscle stimulation—so give it!

On week two, your muscles will be feeling stronger and you may notice that your breathing is better as your cardiovascular system is improving. In preparing to adhere to your program for week two, review your goals. Reflect on what you want to achieve. Focus on the carrot ahead of you, as it is important at this stage to keep your eye on the target and stay hungry for the results you want! Remind yourself of why you started this program and write out your weekly plan and goals for week two.

You will see on your week two workout sheet that I have added three new strength exercises. On your "non-strength days" you should be doing 6 to 10 more minutes of aerobic exercise on each of your three "cardio" training days. Remember to track all your strength and cardio workouts on your workout sheets as this will help you continue the exercises.

"Fit Tip" for Week Two—*Visualization*! Begin to visualize yourself with your health and fitness goals already achieved. Do this when all is quiet and you are alone. Close your eyes and mentally picture yourself the way you ultimately want to look and feel. I like to practice mental imagery when I go to bed. All high level performing athletes use mental visualization to improve their game and perform better. This is a powerful technique to help set you up for success! It's time to believe in yourself; you are getting traction now so keep on keeping on, you got this! 🐾

WEEK TWO EXERCISES

1. Ball Wall Squats
2. Pushups
3. Lat Pulldowns (band)
4. Lunges
5. Standing Chest Press (band)
6. Seated Row (band)
7. **Standing Leg Raise** *
8. **Overhead Press (Light Band)***
9. Step Ups
10. Kneeling Cross Body
11. Plank
12. Ball Abdominal Curls
13. **Ball Abdominal Oblique***

*New exercises in week two

STRENGTH WORKOUT LOG

Week Two

MONDAY		WEDNESDAY		FRIDAY	
Date:		**Date:**		**Date:**	
Warm-up for at least 10 minutes!		*Warm-up for at least 10 minutes!*		*Warm-up for at least 10 minutes!*	
Activity:		Activity:		Activity:	
Minutes:		Minutes:		Minutes:	
Heart Rate:		Heart Rate:		Heart Rate:	
Exercises	Reps	**Exercises**	Reps	**Exercises**	Reps
1. Ball Wall Squats		1. Ball Wall Squats		1. Ball Wall Squats	
2. Push-Ups		2. Push-Ups		2. Push-Ups	
3. Lat Pulldown*		3. Lat Pulldown*		3. Lat Pulldown*	
4. Lunges		4. Lunges		4. Lunges	
5. Standing Chest Press*		5. Standing Chest Press*		5. Standing Chest Press*	
6. Seated Row*		6. Seated Row*		6. Seated Row*	
7. Standing Leg Raise		7. Standing Leg Raise		7. Standing Leg Raise	
8. Overhead Press*		8. Overhead Press*		8. Overhead Press*	
9. Step-Ups		9. Step-Ups		9. Step-Ups	
10. Kneeling Cross Body		10. Kneeling Cross Body		10. Kneeling Cross Body	
11. Plank		11. Plank		11. Plank	
12. Ball Abdominal Curl		12. Ball Abdominal Curl		12. Ball Abdominal Curl	
13. Ball Abdominal Oblique		13. Ball Abdominal Oblique		13. Ball Abdominal Oblique	
STRETCH!		*STRETCH!*		*STRETCH!*	
Weight:		Weight:		Weight:	

These exercises require the use of an exercise band.

CARDIO WORKOUT LOG

Week Two

TUESDAY	THURSDAY	SATURDAY
Date:	**Date:**	**Date:**
Activity:	Activity:	Activity:
Minutes:	Minutes:	Minutes:
Heart Rate:	Heart Rate:	Heart Rate:
Body Weight:	Body Weight:	Body Weight:
Comments:	**Comments:**	**Comments:**
**Remember to stretch at the end of each cardio session!	***Remember to stretch at the end of each cardio session!*	***Remember to stretch at the end of each cardio session!*

Balanced and Whole
Week Two Food

HOW MUCH ARE YOU EATING?

CONGRATULATIONS ON COMPLETING WEEK ONE! By now you're eating primarily whole foods, and getting the hang of planning out your food so you're not caught short—feeling hungry and grabbing the nearest thing...fluffy white bagel, anyone? You've also been logging your food and you have a better idea of what you're eating as well as how much and how often you're eating.

It's not possible, in a general program, to tailor the food quantities to each individual's needs. Needs vary by gender, body size, age and activity level. The Meal Skeleton portion guidelines are meant to be a starting point. Begin with the low end of the serving size range and go up, if you need to, in half-serving intervals. If you're very hungry and/or if your energy is crashing, increase your serving size. If your energy level is stable and you're not starving all the time, you're probably on the right track. Tweak portion sizes and food combinations as you go along based on the information you glean from your food diary. Take note if certain food combinations keep you feeling satisfied for a longer time period.

If your work schedule doesn't allow you to eat regularly, or to eat three meals a day, you can break up your food intake into mini meals. The food plan takes into account one snack per day but you don't need to eat a snack if you're not hungry between meals.

You may need more than one snack if you're eating smaller meals or if there is a long period of time between your meals – that's fine. If you need more than one snack, even if there isn't a long period of time between your meals, that's a sign that you need to change either what you are eating (you may need to eat more fat and/or protein to sustain you longer) and/or how much you are eating (increase portions in ½ serving size intervals). This is the week to experiment with portion sizes and food combinations based on the results you are getting.

In Week One you got rid of all the junk. Your goal in Week Two is to continue to experiment with the "what" and to figure out how much is the "right amount" where you are losing weight and still have plenty of energy for all the fabulous exercise you are now doing!

Throw away your salad bowls!

When it comes to eating the right food proportions, you can fast track your progress by getting rid of your salad bowl. Instead of a big plate of animal food and starchy sides with a small side of veggies and a separate salad, pile those leafy greens right onto your dinner plate. In the dinner plate fraction drawing on page 93, you'll see that the veggies there pull their weight—half the plate, to be exact.

If giving up your salad bowl is making you feel a little deprived, consider having a broth based soup, which can be eaten from that very same bowl! Avoid creamy soups, including soups with "vegetable names" like "Cream of Tomato," if they contain cream, milk, or cheese, and watch the quantity of dense bean or starchy vegetable soups as they should take the place of some or all of your starchy food portions for that meal.

In Week One, you consumed a minimum of 2 servings of vegetables a day. If you didn't consume many vegetables before starting the 21-Day Jumpstart, you're now eating a larger volume of vegetables and have displaced some of the other foods you relied on more heavily, namely starches and animal foods.

Often we only consume a certain volume of food per day and when we add in new foods, like vegetables, we naturally decrease other foods.

This week we are going to literally crowd our plates with veggies by adding in 2 additional servings per day. In week 2, you should be consuming 4 servings of non-starchy vegetables per day. Proceed with caution when consuming raw vegetables if your body is not accustomed to them. Cooking vegetables helps break down the fiber and makes them more digestible. Listen to your body and eat more cooked veggies if your digestive system doesn't handle raw veggies well.

Portions and Proportions!

The size of dinner plates has increased from 9 inches in diameter to 12 inches, on average, for our modern plates. Have you ever tried fitting modern dinner plates into the kitchen cabinets of an older home? They don't fit! Everything has become larger and our perception of portion size is extremely skewed. Consequently, our plate size may look very reasonable to us, when in fact it's just too large. The diameter of our bagels has enjoyed a similar evolution. According to the National Heart Lung and Blood Institute, the average size of a bagel has gone from 3 inches in diameter and 140 calories in 1985 to 6 inches in diameter and 350 calories today[5]. That's the same number of calories as 4 slices of bread!

My husband's daily routine in 1985 consisted of eating a bagel for breakfast most mornings and then not eating again until lunch. If a 20-something, 6 foot 3 inch guy can go from breakfast to lunch on a 1985 bagel, just who are our modern bagels designed for, Sasquatch?!

We have become conditioned to chronically overeat and we feel "empty" when we eat less. This is not necessarily because we have not eaten enough; it is because we are not in touch with our bodies' satiety signals or we don't wait long enough to receive them. We don't eat slowly enough for our stomachs to receive the message from our brain that we have eaten enough. This is why our **Eating Habit Redesign for Week Two** is to eat until you are 2/3 full and wait at least twenty minutes before deciding to eat more.

---

5 http://www.nhlbi.nih.gov/health/educational/wecan/downloads/tip-portion-size.pdf

Most of us are used to eating until we feel physically full—until we feel the fullness in our belly. When we use this as a gauge, we've probably already overeaten. If we've eaten very fast it takes some time, perhaps up to twenty minutes, to feel full or overfull, as the case may be. Just like any other habit, the habit of eating until you feel stuffed can be broken.

At the start of week two, you have already eaten 21 meals consisting of mainly whole foods. You may have eaten larger portions than you needed in week one, but you have already begun the process of becoming reacquainted with your natural hunger and satiety signals. In week two, you will refine this process by stopping before you feel your stomach having to "stretch" to accommodate more food...in other words, by stopping when you're 2/3 full!

Likewise, extend the practice of waiting 20 minutes before eating anything else to the process of deciding whether or not to eat a snack. Instead of choosing to eat a snack, right off the bat, have an eight-ounce glass of water and wait twenty minutes to see if you still feel "hungry."

A lot of my clients tell me that in the afternoon, when they just need "something," having a glass of water works as well as eating a snack or having a cup of coffee.

We are designed to be able to go for four to six hours between meals; eating every two hours is a recent phenomenon. This applies to people who eat three regular meals and do not have health issues that require them to eat more often. If your work schedule forces you to have small "snack-like meals" instead of full meals, you will need to eat more often. Modify when and how you consume daily meal skeleton portions to fit your work schedule, but try eating three meals a day on your days off.

How Hungry are You?

Week two is about tuning in to your body and re-setting the food switch that is driven by habit and not by hunger.

Beginning in week two, every time you eat, rate your hunger on a scale of 0 to 5, where 0 = not hungry at all (still feel "full") and 5 =

over-the-top hungry, i.e. "starving." Record your hunger number on your food log when you record each meal or snack. Try not to let your hunger level reach a five because that's the danger zone when you just need to eat and you don't care what it is. If you know you have a long interval before your next meal, plan ahead and bring a snack. Eat your snack when your hunger is still a four.

Water is essential for optimal health

Water has many benefits besides not containing any calories and by replacing other drinks with water you will reduce your sugar and/or artificial sweetener consumption.

When you're trying to lose weight it's best to eat, and not drink, your calories. Fruit is a whole food (fruit juice is not) and eating fruit is more satisfying than drinking a glass of juice. Lastly, juice has no fiber and fiber is your friend!

Water hydrates our cells and flushes toxins making it important for general health and especially important during weight loss.

In this spirit, we are adding in additional water intake between breakfast and lunch in week two. Aim to consume sixteen to twenty ounces of water between breakfast and lunch.

It is not helpful to consume a lot of water right before or with a meal. A large quantity of water immediately before or with a meal dilutes stomach acid and can hinder digestion. Instead, try to consume your water 20 to 30 minutes before your meal. Drinking sips of water with your meal is fine but don't drink sixteen to twenty ounces with your meal!

Linking water consumption to something you do at regular intervals may to help you remember to drink it. Some of my clients set a timer for 45 minutes before a scheduled meal as a reminder to finish drinking their water. Carrying a canteen helps because it's always with you when you need a sip. Try not to rely on disposable plastic bottles as many contain BPA, a chemical in the plastic that can leach into the water.

If you miss some of your water intake during the day, don't play "catch up" at night; drinking water shortly before bed will result in nighttime waking to use the bathroom, and sleep is also essential to your health! Just try to drink more water the next day.

You may need to drink additional water to replace fluids lost during rigorous exercise, especially in warm weather, since we lose water through perspiration. Water is never limited; the additional water between breakfast and lunch is a minimum, not a maximum. Drink according to your thirst but try to consume the minimum amount of water if you're one of those people who just don't feel thirsty. After more consistent water consumption, many people experience greater thirst.

In week two, portion sizes are limited on starchy foods, animal foods, and added fats. Four servings of vegetables per day are required as a minimum and although fruit is unlimited in week two, fruit cannot be substituted for any of your vegetable servings.

Additionally, if you enjoy eating beans and legumes and can digest them well, add ¼ cup of beans daily in week two. Beans will count as part of your total starch servings. For example, if you include ¼ cup of beans, decrease your starchy foods serving in that meal by ¼ cup. The *Week Two at a Glance* section contains all these changes.

If you're not cooking your own meals, you should have already scoped out ways to get your vegetable servings during Week One. You can include raw vegetables as snacks or as part of meals. Prepping (cleaning and cutting) vegetables for the week will become a crucial part of your Sunday as you look to eat twice as many vegetables as you did in week one...being prepared saves you from the "unhealthy grab" every time!

WEEK TWO AT A GLANCE

Week two builds on week one...

Do everything you did in week one and add the following...

- **Water:** Add an additional 16-20 ounces of water between breakfast and lunch. Don't consume your water less than 20 to 30 minutes before lunch. It is fine to sip water with lunch or dinner but don't drink large quantities of water with your meals.

- **Coffee or Tea:** If you drink more than one cup per day, try to have your second cup after lunch so it doesn't interfere with your hunger signals.

- **Vegetables:** 4 servings daily. Beginning in week two, add an additional 2 servings of non-starchy vegetables per day. One serving= ½ cup of cooked vegetables (including cooked leafy greens) or raw "chunky" vegetables or 1 cup of raw leafy greens.

- **Limit portion sizes on animal foods:** An average serving of animal food is about 4 ounces. Smaller women may do well on 3 ounces and larger men may need to go up to eating 5 or 6 ounces. It also depends on the type of animal food—for a fatty fish, like salmon, 3 oz. goes a long way; whereas with leaner foods, like poultry breast meat, a larger serving size might be required. Have a maximum of 3 servings per day of animal foods. Eggs count as a serving of animal food, the average serving size is 2 eggs.

- **Dairy:** Continue to observe portion limits. Do not exceed 4 "wedges" per day. Dairy can be optionally used as part of meals or as a snack. There is no minimum for dairy.

- **Limit portion sizes on starchy foods**: Limit servings of starchy foods (potatoes, winter squash, roots and tubers, corn, beans and grains) to 3 servings per day if eating animal foods. If not eating any animal foods *the entire day*, limit servings of starchy foods to 6 servings. Try to alternate between grains, starchy vegetables, and beans each day.

Serving Size Ranges for <u>Cooked</u> Starchy Foods:

Corn: Women= ½ - ¾ cup, Men= ¾ - 1 cup

Winter Squash: Women= 1 – 1 ½ cups, Men=1 ½- 2 cups

Yams, all potatoes and Jerusalem Artichokes:
Women= 1, 5-inch potato (4 oz.) or ½ larger potato or ½ cup mashed or 3/4 - 1 cup cubes or slices. Men=1, 7-inch potato (6oz.) or ¾ cup mashed or 1 – 1-1/4 cup cubes or slices. Try to eat white potatoes roasted/baked with skin on. **Note:** Cassava (yuca, manioc) and taro are starchy vegetables. Cassava and taro must be cooked as they are toxic when consumed raw. If you know how to properly prepare them, the serving size for taro is 25% less (¾ the size) than a serving of potatoes; for cassava/yuca, serving size is 50% less (½ the size of a serving of potatoes).

Grains: Rice, Quinoa, Farro, Barley, Wheat, Spelt, Kamut, Rye:
Women= ½-¾ cup, Men= ¾-1 cup

Grains: Oats, Kasha, Bulgur: Women= ¾-1 cup, Men= 1-1 ¼ cups

Bread: 1-2 slices (unisex)

- **Beans**: Include ¼ cup per day, if you digest them well. Some people who don't digest beans well can eat peas, green beans, edamame and/or lentils, mung or adzuki. If beans agree with you, ½ cup is a full serving size.

- **Limit portion sizes on added fats**: Limit added fats from butter or oils, to max of 2 tbsp. per day.

DINNER PLATE FRACTIONS...EASY VISUAL PORTION SIZES!

Week two calls for increasing your portions of vegetables while limiting your portions of almost everything else.

While portion sizes are given in cups or ounces, if you aren't cooking your own food or aren't measuring it with a food scale and/or measuring cups, an easy way to see if your meal proportions are roughly correct is to use the recommended fractions below.

¼ of your plate should be for animal foods
¼ of your plate should be for starchy foods
½ of your plate should be for non-starchy vegetables

If you are eating in a restaurant and the portion of animal protein you are served takes up more than a quarter of your plate, chances are it is an oversized portion. Cut it in half and remove it to another plate to take home. Use the same method for starchy foods. Order salad dressing on the side and use 2 tbsp. of dressing or no more than 1-2 tsp. of extra-virgin olive oil and/or as much vinegar as you would like.

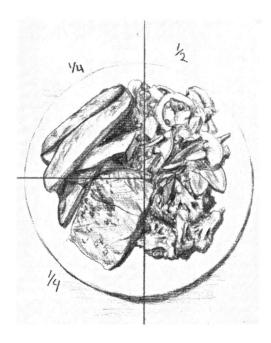

Week Two Daily Meal Skeleton

FIRST MORNING WATER

BREAKFAST

Whole Fruit

Choice of Food

1 oz. nuts daily max if eating animal protein
Additional water between breakfast and lunch

LUNCH/DINNER*

2 servings of vegetables

1 serving animal protein (poultry, fish, meat, eggs, dairy)

with optional 1 serving whole grain or starchy vegetable (never both) OR

Grain & Bean Combo OR

Starchy Vegetable & Bean Combo OR

Grain & Nuts or Seeds Combo OR

Starchy Vegetables & Nuts or Seeds Combo

* Lunch and Dinner have the same food choices/Choices are per meal

Eating Habit Redesign: Wait 20 minutes before eating seconds.

WEEK TWO DAILY MEAL SKELETON GUIDELINES

- Add 16–20 ounces of water between breakfast and lunch; finish drinking at least 20 minutes before eating lunch.

- Add an additional 2 servings of non-starchy vegetables per day bringing the minimum to 4 servings daily. One serving= ½ cup of cooked vegetables (including cooked leafy greens) or raw "chunky" vegetables or 1 cup of raw leafy greens.

- Add ¼ cup of beans (if you digest them well) to one of your daily meals or enjoy as snack.

- If eating animal foods, limit nuts to no more than one, 1 oz. serving per day. Nut butters count toward nut servings. A full portion of nut butter is 2 tbsp. For example, if you have 2 tbsp. of peanut or almond butter in one meal, you can't have any other nuts/seeds in meals or snacks; if you have 1 tbsp. of nut butter you can also have ½ oz. of nuts.

Week Two Food Diary

Date_____

First AM Water

Dairy

Water between Breakfast & Lunch

TIME	AMOUNT	FOOD/BEVERAGE	SAT DOWN? Y/N	HUNGER RATING (0–5)

What went well? _____

Struggles? _____

What to do differently tomorrow? _____

Week Two Food Diary

Date_____

First AM Water

Dairy

Water between Breakfast & Lunch

TIME	AMOUNT	FOOD/BEVERAGE	SAT DOWN? Y/N	HUNGER RATING (0-5)

What went well? _____

Struggles? _____

What to do differently tomorrow? _____

Week Two Food Diary

Date_____

First AM Water

Dairy

Water between Breakfast & Lunch

TIME	AMOUNT	FOOD/BEVERAGE	SAT DOWN? Y/N	HUNGER RATING (0–5)

What went well? _____

Struggles? _____

What to do differently tomorrow? _____

Week Two Food Diary

Date_____

First AM Water

Water between Breakfast & Lunch

Dairy

TIME	AMOUNT	FOOD/BEVERAGE	SAT DOWN? Y/N	HUNGER RATING (0-5)

What went well? _____

Struggles? _____

What to do differently tomorrow? _____

Week Two Food Diary

Date_____

First AM Water

Dairy

Water between Breakfast & Lunch

TIME	AMOUNT	FOOD/BEVERAGE	SAT DOWN? Y/N	HUNGER RATING (0-5)

What went well? _____

Struggles? _____

What to do differently tomorrow? _____

Week Two Food Diary

Date_____

First AM Water

Dairy

Water between Breakfast & Lunch

TIME	AMOUNT	FOOD/BEVERAGE	SAT DOWN? Y/N	HUNGER RATING (0-5)

What went well? _____

Struggles? _____

What to do differently tomorrow? _____

Week Two Food Diary

Date_____

First AM Water

Dairy

Water between Breakfast & Lunch

TIME	AMOUNT	FOOD/BEVERAGE	SAT DOWN? Y/N	HUNGER RATING (0-5)

What went well? _____

Struggles? _____

What to do differently tomorrow? _____

21-Day Jumpstart Food and Exercise Journal
Week Two

____ / ____ / ____ — ____ / ____ / ____

Please log your feelings, thoughts, and comments on how your daily nutrition and exercise has been going during week two.

_____

_____

_____

_____

_____

_____

_____

_____

_____

_____

_____

_____

_____

_____

_____

_____

_____

_____

_____

_____

Balanced and Whole
Week Three Exercise

JUMP-STARTING WEEK THREE EXERCISE

GREAT JOB, YOU ARE 14 days in—you are doing an awesome job! You are two-thirds done...rounding third and heading for home! Your body is now getting used to exercise. Things are starting to get easier so you may need to step up the intensity a bit. By now you should really be pushing your strength exercises so you are bringing your muscles (slowly and safely) to what is called momentary muscle fatigue. This is when you can't perform another repetition in good form, or what is referred to as "maxing out" on that strength exercise.

Listed on the week three strength workout sheet are two additional new exercises, rounding your strength routine out to 15 total exercises. Your aerobic workout should now be up to at least 20 minutes of continuous movement in your target heart rate zone. This is a good time to again review and reflect on your short-term and long-term goals. You need to stay disciplined and challenge yourself to stay on course and keep working on the strong foundation you are building. Nothing is going to stop you now—you are going to complete this! Plan and write out your weekly workout schedule in your planner, calendar or phone. Record your specific game plan: Walk—Mon., Wed. and Fri. 6 AM; Strength Train—Tues., Thurs. and Sat. 5:30 PM; Sun. rest; Repeat.

Your Fit Tip for Week Three is—*Give Yourself Positive Reinforcement!* Think of something you can reward yourself with for completing the 21 days....something pretty big that you will look forward to doing.

Maybe dinner out at a nice restaurant, some new exercise clothes, one of those fit-bits for tracking your progress, a massage...something you have wanted that will help reinforce your commitment to yourself. Looking forward to this treat or reward upon completion will help keep you on course. Besides, you have sacrificed a lot, you are making major positive changes; you are worth it and deserve it!

WEEK THREE EXERCISES

1. Ball Wall Squats
2. Push ups
3. Lat Pulldowns (band)
4. Lunges
5. Standing Chest Press (band)
6. Seated Row (band)
7. Standing Leg raise
8. **Chest Flys (band)***
9. Overhead Press (light band)
10. Step Ups
11. **Bicep Curls (band)***
12. Kneeling Cross Body
13. Plank
14. Ball Abdominal Curl
15. Ball Abdominal Oblique

*New exercises in week three

STRENGTH WORKOUT LOG

Week Three

MONDAY		WEDNESDAY		FRIDAY	
Date:		**Date:**		**Date:**	
Warm-up for at least 10 minutes!		*Warm-up for at least 10 minutes!*		*Warm-up for at least 10 minutes!*	
Activity:		Activity:		Activity:	
Minutes:		Minutes:		Minutes:	
Heart Rate:		Heart Rate:		Heart Rate:	
Exercises	Reps	**Exercises**	Reps	**Exercises**	Reps
1. Ball Wall Squats		1. Ball Wall Squats		1. Ball Wall Squats	
2. Push-Ups		2. Push-Ups		2. Push-Ups	
3. Lat Pulldown*		3. Lat Pulldown*		3. Lat Pulldown*	
4. Lunges		4. Lunges		4. Lunges	
5. Standing Chest Press*		5. Standing Chest Press*		5. Standing Chest Press*	
6. Seated Row*		6. Seated Row*		6. Seated Row*	
7. Standing Leg Raise		7. Standing Leg Raise		7. Standing Leg Raise	
8. Chest Flys*		8. Chest Flys*		8. Chest Flys*	
9. Overhead Press*		9. Overhead Press*		9. Overhead Press*	
10. Step-Ups		10. Step-Ups		10. Step-Ups	
11. Bicep Curls*		11. Bicep Curls*		11. Bicep Curls*	
12. Kneeling Cross Body		12. Kneeling Cross Body		12. Kneeling Cross Body	
13. Plank		13. Plank		13. Plank	
14. Ball Abdominal Curl		14. Ball Abdominal Curl		14. Ball Abdominal Curl	
15. Ball Abdominal Oblique		15. Ball Abdominal Oblique		15. Ball Abdominal Oblique	
STRETCH!		*STRETCH!*		*STRETCH!*	
Weight:		Weight:		Weight:	

*These exercises require the use of an exercise band.

CARDIO WORKOUT LOG

Week Three

TUESDAY	THURSDAY	SATURDAY
Date:	**Date:**	**Date:**
Activity:	Activity:	Activity:
Minutes:	Minutes:	Minutes:
Heart Rate:	Heart Rate:	Heart Rate:
Body Weight:	Body Weight:	Body Weight:
Comments:	**Comments:**	**Comments:**
**Remember to stretch at the end of each cardio session!	***Remember to stretch at the end of each cardio session!*	***Remember to stretch at the end of each cardio session!*

NEXT STEPS

Congratulations, you did it! You took on the challenge and achieved it... great job on laying down an excellent foundation and starting some new, very healthy habits! You have experienced what it means to put it all together with whole-food eating and regular exercise, and have jump-started your body towards better health! So now you may be asking, what's next?

Exercise Your Potential—Keep it Fresh and Boost the Intensity:

Exercise is a way of life and you have just begun to make it part of your weekly routine. Here are a few tips for increasing the intensity of your strength and cardio exercise to continue to make more progress and gain additional benefits.

Intensifying Your Strength Training

- Perform more repetitions with your exercises but keep the reps slow! If you are easily getting 20 repetitions with the exercise bands you are using, increase the thickness of the bands to make the repetition more difficult.

- **Push Ups**—If you haven't tried pushups from your toes then go for it! Try to see how many of these you can do then break it down to your knees.

  If you are doing your pushups on your toes, challenge yourself for more reps. To intensify your pushups even further, go slower and go lower trying to touch your nose to the ground.

- **Plank**—If you have been doing your plank from your knees and haven't gotten up to your elbows and toes yet, try raising up to your elbows for as long as you can and then break it down to your knees. If you have been doing your plank exercises from your elbows and toes then increase the time. Try mixing in a side plank with your forward plank. Alternate side and forward plank, holding each position for 10 to 15 seconds. Advance to what I call

"Plank-Ups" where you start at a plank on your elbows and toes, then move to a pushup position and drop back down to the elbow plank position, continuously alternating these two positions for a minute.

Variety

- Investigate using a **nylon strap suspension system.** This is a strap exercise kit that you can simply put into a doorway like your exercise bands or cinch up on a hook or hang over a bar such as a swing set and do an entire body workout with it. It comes with directions and an instruction manual. One such apparatus is the TRX® Suspension Training. Go to www.TRXtraining.com. Oftentimes during the week when I have an hour break between clients, I will go to a nearby park, or maybe I will be at home, either way, I like to hook up my suspension system and get in a good 30-minute total body workout.

- **Dumbbells**—Step up your strength training workout routine by mixing in dumbbells. If you have never used dumbbells before then you need to do your homework and research this equipment. It's best to work out with a partner when using dumbbells. If you have used dumbbells before, then follow the workout guidelines I have provided here, going largest to smallest muscle groups and do one set, maintaining the 15 to 20 repetitions range.

- **Circuit Training**—"Amp up" your workouts with Circuit Training. Combine cardio in your strength workouts by interspersing intervals of cardio exercise with every two strength exercises. Start with 30 seconds to a minute then increase your cardio intervals to 2 minutes. Good cardio intervals are jumping jacks, skipping rope, jogging on and off a step, kickboxing on a heavy bag, stationary biking, walking or jogging on a treadmill, or using an elliptical machine.

- **Use a Personal Trainer**—Consider hiring a nationally certified personal trainer, even if you use them only to coach you once a week. They will guide you through safe exercises, give you variety, keep it fresh and challenge you more than you will do on your own to help bring you to the next level. Consider doing "partner training" with a buddy and split the cost of the trainer with a friend.

Intensifying Your Cardio Days

- **Increase Your Speed**: As your cardiovascular endurance gets better and your cardio exercise gets easier to do, try to go further in the same 30-minute time. Pick up your walking or jogging pace, training in the upper range of your target heart rate zone.

- **Jog**: If you haven't tried to jog yet, try adding in some light jogging intervals. Start with 30 seconds and then work up to 2 min. or more of jogging intervals in between your brisk walking. Before you know it you will be able to jog continuously for much longer periods of time. Make sure you have a good pair of running shoes to absorb the impact.

- **Register for a Road Race**: Consider going into a 5k walk or road race. Set a goal to train for a 5k even if you are going to walk it. Once you have experienced one of these events, the group energy of a 5k will motivate you to do more.

- **Variety**: Change it up! If you have been only walking, consider mixing in some other form of cardio such as biking, hiking, swimming, or using an elliptical machine. The variation will keep it fresh, train different muscles and make the exercises a little more challenging on your cardiovascular system. Plus, you may end up burning more calories!

- **Buddy up**: Exercise with a friend who you know is an avid walker or jogger and will challenge you to step up your pace and distance.

Staying Consistent

In order for your habits to stick long term, your next step involves consistency. Here are some key points and reminders to help you stay on track and get you to the next level:

Exercise Reminders for Success
- List your long-term (one-year), intermediate (6-month) and short-term (3-month) goals.
- Plan your week and write in exercise on your schedule, planner, or in your phone.
- Set out your workout clothes the night before.
- Gradually work up to 30 minutes of daily activity and take one day off per week.
- Alternate strength and cardio days.
- Always warm up on your strength days, perform each exercise slowly, but move quickly with little rest between strength exercises to gain more cardiovascular benefits.
- Stretch after every cardio and strength workout.
- On cardio days exercise in your target heart rate zone (refer to the target HR chart in Appendix D)

Tips to Keep On Keeping On:
- Get good quality, uninterrupted sleep.
- Post your goals where you can see them.
- Exercise with a partner or good friend who is serious about long-term wellness.
- Gear up—treat yourself to quality sneakers or workout attire to motivate you.
- Create a fun and inviting exercise environment: listen to your favorite music, put on an enjoyable TV show or the news, set up an appealing and welcoming room to workout in.
- Hire a certified personal trainer.

- If you fall off the healthy eating or exercise path for a couple days, don't beat yourself up, it's ok. Just get back on the path and remember you are in it for the long haul!
- Simply tell yourself to begin. **Some days the desire to exercise may be low, and it can be tough to get started**. But once you get those workout clothes and sneakers on, and initiate the process, the hardest part is over and it gets easier as you go.

Believe in yourself. The body is amazing and you can transform it into whatever you desire. Develop a daily affirmation and repeat it every morning. This is powerful. Develop your own, but it could be something like, *"I am strong, vibrant, happy, beautiful, positive and balanced and can achieve anything I desire!"*

Balanced and Whole
Week Three Food

REFINING THE WHAT & THE HOW MUCH

CONGRATULATIONS ON COMPLETING 14 DAYS of your 21-Day Jumpstart! Do something to celebrate that doesn't involve sugar or alcohol! See a movie (sans popcorn), go hiking or grab coffee with a friend...anything that feels like a reward.

Regardless of whether or not you followed your plan to the letter, if you kept your food diary and paid attention to your body's cues, you likely have a lot more information about your relationship with food than you did when you started. Perhaps these two weeks have confirmed some things you already knew but haven't acted on. Since embarking on the 21-Day Jumpstart you've had to shift more of your mental focus towards your food and exercise habits, but this time commitment will decrease as you develop systems to simplify your daily routines. Planning your food for the week, including purchasing and prepping, takes a while to come together but as it becomes a habit, it requires less effort.

Whether or not you have lost weight in the first 14 days, if you followed the program, you have drastically reduced your consumption of added sugars and eliminated almost all processed foods.

You have also increased the amount of vegetables and fruit that you consume daily, thus increasing your intake of vitamins, minerals, phytonutrients and fiber. These are huge positive dietary changes!

Changes like these usually take much longer than 2 weeks to implement. If you have been able to do it, then you have already proved that you can do it. And you can continue to do it in Week Three and beyond...it all comes down to your choices!

Should we eat the same amount of food every day?

We're not robots, although it would be easier to eat like one! Our energy level and hunger fluctuate daily. Why, then, do we think we should eat the same amount of food every day?

If you chronically overate before starting the 21-Day Jumpstart, it will likely take time for you to feel satisfied with less food. You have begun that process after 21 meals of eating consistently smaller portions during week two.

This doesn't mean that you will not experience differing hunger levels on different days. Eating a varied amount of food daily keeps our metabolism from slowing down due to consistently reduced calorie consumption... and this mirrors nature.

One of the most important goals of the 21-Day Jumpstart is to learn how to tune in to your body's hunger cues. Is that urge to eat due to boredom, loneliness, or physical hunger? Beginning in Week Two you were recording your hunger number in your food diary. If you're doing that, you can decide not to eat if your hunger level is three or below, especially if it is the evening and you will be going to sleep before your hunger becomes a four.

The hungry days...

When we have one of those hungry days it helps to try parsing out the cause of the hunger: Ask yourself, is it physical or emotional? Stress drives hunger as does rigorous and prolonged physical exercise, fatigue and hormonal fluctuations. These variations are normal and they won't disappear because you are following the 21-Day Jumpstart. Different reasons for increased hunger need to be addressed in different ways.

And hungry nights!

One of the most challenging times of day is the evening from after dinner until bedtime. There isn't a magic bullet to stop nighttime eating—what you can do is to eliminate the triggers in your environment (don't watch TV if you always snack while watching) and the triggers in your pantry (get rid of the food that "calls" to you at night!) and create as many deterrents to nighttime eating as possible! That brings us to the **Eating Habit Redesign for Week Three**: Brush your teeth immediately after dinner. By brushing your teeth early you "close your mouth" for the evening the way some moms close the kitchen when their children are little...you have to be your own mom...close your mouth (to food!) and put yourself to bed earlier!

Manage your stress!

Finding nonfood ways to relieve stress will help you stop turning to sugar as a quick stress buster. Stress is part of our daily landscape and the best way to cope is to learn to manage it.

Just taking a few deep and slow breaths often does the trick. Practice deep breathing every evening of week three so you can add this technique to your stress-reducing toolbox.

Lie flat and put your hand on your belly. Breathe deeply and slowly until you can feel your hand being pushed up when you inhale and dropping when you exhale. Deep breathing should be done slowly. You can (silently) count out the inhale, count a brief hold and then count the exhale, drawing it out as long as possible. When you start you may only be able to make it last for 3 counts of 5 but you can gradually work your way up to higher counts...with practice you should be able to work your way up to 30 seconds (3 counts of 10) for one complete breath.

Find Your Fix

When we're experiencing internal stress, we sometimes feel that if the people around us would only change their behavior we would feel better. It just doesn't work this way and the sooner we accept it, the better we become at developing coping mechanisms.

I can't say enough about how effective deep breathing is. Anything medical, no matter how routine, stresses me out and going into deep breathing mode is how I cope.

Inevitably the staff will ask me if I'm a runner, because the breathing makes my heart rate so slow! This technique is truly amazing, but it can only work for you if you use it.

If breathing just isn't your thing, you need to find a fix that works for you. Recently, a client of mine, who is a grandma, told me she started playing Candy Crush on her phone while waiting for her husband, who is perpetually late. She used to get stressed out waiting for him and now the time flies by because she's playing on her phone. Problem solved! Incorporate as many fixes as you need for the routine stressors in your life but remember, you can only "fix" yourself.

Sometimes you just need more food!

On days when you do prolonged and more strenuous exercise you will need to eat more. I have found that most women eat more the week before their moon cycle (week before moon cycle = voracious appetite) and then their appetite drops off with the arrival of their period. From a weight perspective, the two weeks typically balance each other out. Since this is a three week program, where you are in your cycle may affect your weight changes...don't let that stop you from eating more the week before your period. You should be listening to your body's cues, not ignoring them! What you eat more of, however, may be what you will want to change!

The Broccoli Method

I'm always amazed by people's creativity in developing strategies that work for them. All you need is the mindset that you know your own body best. My favorite case: The Broccoli Lady. She wanted to lose weight after having her last baby. She was cooking and eating meals with her children, and had tried, unsuccessfully, to eat less at dinner time.

Her solution? She cooked broccoli and ate it, a lot of it, before sitting down to dinner with her family. When she did sit down to eat dinner, she already felt "full" from the broccoli so she ate less and started losing weight. She lost all her baby weight this way! Now, I'm not suggesting that you try this approach, and use your two extra vegetable servings to eat broccoli before dinner—that's just crazy, isn't it?!

I must admit that I love broccoli, and I've been told by my family that I serve it a bit too often. A while back my son, Willie, went on a broccoli strike. So, if you're like Willie (or George H. W. Bush), this is the worst idea you've ever heard of, but that's the point...one strategy doesn't fit all, so master the mindset and think outside the broccoli!

Two steps forward, one step back...

Change is never linear. It can be frustrating but hang in there and you will start to feel more and more in control as you begin to cement your healthier habits. You never "arrive" at the destination, meaning that you can eat as much as you want and not gain any weight (that's only in our dreams). There will always be times when you don't make stellar choices but you can adjust at the very next meal. If you eat a lot at one meal, eat a little less at the next—feast then famine—which is the natural rhythm of life.

Stop thinking in terms of tomorrow, next Monday or next month. Stop thinking about when you have more time, when your life calms down, or when you have a Fairy Godmother...you've already started, so just keep swimming (remember Dory?)!

Who said it was fair?

My husband has been telling my kids that life isn't fair since they were in preschool. As a health counselor, I see great value in internalizing this principle at a very young age. The truth is that based on our individual genetics, we will be able to eat differing amounts and types of food, while still maintaining our weight and our health. And this is a moving target. But there are still heaps we can do to increase our quality of life by making healthier choices.

We are dynamic creatures. What works at age 30 may not work at 40, 50, or 60. One thing is for certain, though, we need to eat well and move our bodies. Strength training is the only way to maintain and build lean muscle as we age. Whether you rearrange the furniture in your house every other day, use resistance and your own body weight as you've done for the past 14 days, or lift weights at the gym, once you hit 40 you can't keep fit without doing something anymore.

Our muscles are the "engines" of our metabolism. Exercise reshapes our body by changing our body composition (percentage of fat and muscle). And being stronger greatly improves the quality of our life as we age.

What do you want to be able to do when you're 80? Put it on a *Post-it*® note where you can see it every day. This is the big picture and achieving it is more important than a number on the scale.

Two people can weigh the same while looking and feeling very differently based on their body composition. It's not just changes in your weight that make a difference; looking better in your sleeveless shirt is a big bonus too!

Have a realistic body image!

It's important to have a realistic ideal body image based on your body type. If you are not built long and willowy no amount of calorie restriction and exercise will transform your body into that form. If you have to do extreme long-term calorie restriction to maintain your goal weight, it's not a good goal weight for you.

Love yourself more!

Regardless of our age, many of us have not learned to love ourselves because we have an unrealistic ideal or have struggled with lifelong feelings of guilt, fear and shame related to food and our bodies. When you indulge in a "treat," do your best to make it a conscious choice, free of guilt, fear and shame. We shall overcome!

The best action you can take for your health is deciding on your goal and consistently moving forward on that course. It is possible to achieve a balance between the right amount of food and the right amount of exercise.

It's a process that you've already begun with the 21-Day Jumpstart. The weeks beyond these first three will include seeking out that balance and making healthy choices most of the time while having an occasional treat—and it's not a "cheat!" Remember, you aren't going for perfect, just go for good enough!

WEEK THREE AT A GLANCE

Week Three builds on Weeks One and Two...

Do everything you did in Weeks One and Two and add the following:

- **Water:** Add an additional 16-20 ounces of water between lunch and dinner. Don't consume your water less than 20 to 30 minutes before dinner. It is fine to have sips of water with dinner but don't drink large quantities of water with your meals.

- **Vegetables:** 6 servings daily during week three, so you need to add 2 additional servings of non-starchy vegetables per day to bring your daily total up to 6 servings. One serving= ½ cup of cooked vegetables (including cooked leafy greens) or raw "chunky" vegetables or 1 cup of raw leafy greens.

- **Fruit:** Limit fruit to 2 whole fruits a day or the equivalent. For berries, cherries, grapes and all fruits too large to consume whole, use one cup as a serving size.

- **Beans:** Include ½ cup per day, if you digest them well.

Week Three Daily Meal Skeleton

FIRST MORNING WATER

BREAKFAST
Whole Fruit

Choice of Food

+ 2 additional servings of veggies • 2 whole fruits daily max
Water between breakfast and lunch & between lunch and dinner

LUNCH/DINNER*

2 servings of vegetables

1 serving animal protein (poultry, fish, meat, eggs, dairy)

with optional 1 serving whole grain or starchy vegetable (never both) OR

Grain & Bean Combo OR

Starchy Vegetable & Bean Combo OR

Grain & Nuts or Seeds Combo OR

Starchy Vegetables & Nuts or Seeds Combo

* Lunch and Dinner have the same food choices/Choices are per meal

Eating Habit Redesign: Brush your teeth immediately after dinner.

WEEK THREE DAILY MEAL SKELETON GUIDELINES

- Add 16–20 ounces of water between lunch and dinner, and finish drinking at least 20 minutes before eating dinner.

- Add an additional 2 servings of non-starchy vegetables per day, bringing the minimum to 6 servings daily. You can add the vegetable servings to any of your meals or use as snacks. One serving= ½ cup of cooked vegetables (including cooked leafy greens) or raw "chunky" vegetables or 1 cup of raw leafy greens.

- Increase beans to ½ cup daily—use as part of one or more daily meals or as snack.

- Limit fruit to two whole fruits or equivalent per day.

Week Three Food Diary

Date_____

First AM Water

Water between Breakfast & Lunch

Dairy

Water between Lunch & Dinner

TIME	AMOUNT	FOOD/BEVERAGE	SAT DOWN? Y/N	HUNGER RATING (0-5)

What went well? _____

Struggles? _____

What to do differently tomorrow? _____

Week Three Food Diary

Date_____

First AM Water

Water between Breakfast & Lunch

Dairy

Water between Lunch & Dinner

TIME	AMOUNT	FOOD/BEVERAGE	SAT DOWN? Y/N	HUNGER RATING (0-5)

What went well? _____

Struggles? _____

What to do differently tomorrow? _____

Week Three Food Diary

Date_____

First AM Water

Water between Breakfast & Lunch

Dairy

Water between Lunch & Dinner

TIME	AMOUNT	FOOD/BEVERAGE	SAT DOWN? Y/N	HUNGER RATING (0-5)

What went well? _____

Struggles? _____

What to do differently tomorrow? _____

Week Three Food Diary

Date_____

First AM Water

Water between Breakfast & Lunch

Dairy

Water between Lunch & Dinner

TIME	AMOUNT	FOOD/BEVERAGE	SAT DOWN? Y/N	HUNGER RATING (0-5)

What went well? _____

Struggles? _____

What to do differently tomorrow? _____

Week Three Food Diary

Date_____

First AM Water

Water between Breakfast & Lunch

Dairy

Water between Lunch & Dinner

TIME	AMOUNT	FOOD/BEVERAGE	SAT DOWN? Y/N	HUNGER RATING (0-5)

What went well? _____

Struggles? _____

What to do differently tomorrow? _____

Week Three Food Diary

Date_____

First AM Water

Water between Breakfast & Lunch

Dairy

Water between Lunch & Dinner

TIME	AMOUNT	FOOD/BEVERAGE	SAT DOWN? Y/N	HUNGER RATING (0-5)

What went well? _____

Struggles? _____

What to do differently tomorrow?_____

Week Three Food Diary

Date_____

First AM Water   Water between Breakfast & Lunch

Dairy   Water between Lunch & Dinner

TIME	AMOUNT	FOOD/BEVERAGE	SAT DOWN? Y/N	HUNGER RATING (0-5)

What went well? _____

Struggles? _____

What to do differently tomorrow?_____

21-Day Jumpstart Food and Exercise Journal
Week Three

____ / ____ / ____ — ____ / ____ / ____

Please log your feelings, thoughts, and comments on how your daily nutrition and exercise has been going during week three.

_____

_____

_____

_____

_____

_____

_____

_____

_____

_____

_____

_____

_____

_____

_____

_____

_____

_____

_____

_____

_____

BEYOND WEEK THREE—BACK TO BASICS

You've completed the 21-Day Jumpstart—Hooray for you! If you stick with the basics of the program you will be well positioned to accomplish your goals, whether you're trying to lose more weight or to maintain your current weight.

THE BASICS OF WHAT

Eat your Vegetables!

- If you had to work hard to eat six servings of vegetables and two whole fruits per day in Week Three, keep it going! If you continue to consume more vegetables and fruits you will be naturally consuming less of everything else.

Reduce Added Sugars

- Reduce flour-based products with added sugars (cookies, cake, muffins, scones, sweets, etc.)

- Eliminate flavored yogurt—you did it for 21 Days...so continue to stick with plain!

- Avoid condiments that are high in sugar like ketchup, barbeque sauces, salad dressings, etc.

- Read labels carefully. Watch out for "health foods" like granola, bars, and nutritional shake mixes, etc.; these can also be high in sugar.

- Beware of coffee "drinks" and smoothies...most are high in sugar!

- Eat whole fruit instead of drinking fruit juice. Juice is higher in sugar than a piece of whole fruit and juice doesn't contain any fiber. Eating fruit is more satisfying!

- Eliminate all artificial sweeteners!

Reduce Flour/Pulverized Grain

- Reduce "filler" foods like bagels, pizza, bread, rolls, etc. Be deliberate about when you choose to eat them.

- Snack on whole foods like fruits, vegetables, nuts, seeds and legumes instead of flour-based snacks like pretzels and chips.

Choose Quality Fats

- Read the ingredients list on food labels (not just the nutrition info) and never purchase foods containing hydrogenated oils. Expeller-pressed, organic, unrefined oils are best.

- Make unrefined extra virgin olive oil your "go-to" oil for everything except high heat cooking.

- Remember that whole foods like avocados, olives, nuts and seeds are good sources of healthy fats.

Drink water...lots of it!

THE BASICS OF HOW MUCH

Mind portion sizes!

- Use dinner plate fractions for easy portion control.

- Alternate between grains and starchy vegetables and don't consume both in a meal containing animal protein (except on Thanksgiving!).

- Try to eat ½ cup of beans most days, if possible...it will keep your fiber consumption up, which reduces your calorie consumption naturally.

- Portion out fats, like dressings, sauces and nut butters, with a measuring tablespoon and put 1 oz. of nuts into baggies; eat one baggie a day.

- Many restaurants serve oversized portions of animal foods, so eat half and take the rest home.

Vegetables:

- When planning meals, focus on vegetables first and animal foods second. If vegetables aren't an afterthought you're less likely to let them "slip."

EATING HABIT REDESIGNS—THE BASIC 3!

1. Sit down when you eat anything!
2. Eat until you are 2/3 full and wait at least twenty minutes before deciding to eat more.
3. Brush your teeth immediately after dinner.

THE BASICS OF SUCCESS

- **Avoid your triggers!** Use what you've learned through your food diary; identify your trigger foods and avoid them. Avoid trigger people, places and activities too, if possible! For example, if you always eat in front of the TV, don't watch TV for a while or force yourself to get up and sit in your kitchen for a nighttime snack... if you must snack!

- If you just need "something," try a warm cup of herbal tea with a tsp. of raw honey or a mug of warm water instead of a snack in the evenings.

- Ask your wait person not to bring bread to the table when you dine in restaurants—avoiding temptation is better than being more disciplined!

- Preparing your own foods is the best way to control the quality and quantity of the fats in your diet.

- Seek non-food ways to go to your happy place...listen to great music, take a hot bath, make love, phone a friend, and if all else fails—go to bed earlier!

- Be cautious with coffee and alcohol use; try not to rely on them to wind up and wind down.

Transition from Bill

"It is a whole lot cheaper and easier to maintain good health through proper exercise, diet and emotional balance than to regain it once it is lost."
— Dr. Kenneth Cooper

Balancing it all out and feeling whole...

Now that you have achieved the 21-day jumpstart, let's take a look further ahead at the big picture; obtaining the long-term rewards—reaping the "harvest" from the seeds you have planted. I'm not just referring to the many health benefits that you will be enjoying from your new healthy habits, **by continuing on this path, you can transform your life to become a more balanced person.** As author Rabbi Karyn D. Kedar says in her Balance Poem reprinted on page 11, "Strive for an equal balance of all the parts" for balance in mind, body and soul!

Life is a balancing act. By nature we are meant to be in balance. Our lives are so busy and full of activities that pull us out of balance. Trying to balance work and play hours, family time, social time and alone time, sleep and rest time....how do you balance it all and stay happy and fulfilled? It is our belief that by exercising regularly and fueling our bodies with healthy, whole food nutrition, we can keep our systems performing optimally and our bodies, minds and spirits, in balance.

Julie has built in balance for you with your 21-day food plan so you are getting the excellent nutrition your body needs, and I have created balance within your exercise program with 3 days of cardio and 3 days of strength. I have designed body balance within the exercises incorporating lower body and upper body movements, opposing anterior and posterior muscle work and exercise exertion balanced with stretching and rest.

It's a Way of Life Mentality

Now that you know you can commit to this whole food and exercise program for 21 days, adopt the attitude that you can do this for life. Have the mindset that this isn't just a short-term weight loss fix, rather a healthy way of life. The mindset that you will STAY at a favorable body weight and enjoy the many benefits from the positive habits you have initiated for good...isn't that what you want? Staying fit and healthy is a process. Every week you can improve upon what you have done. The longer you stay on course with eating healthy and exercising, the more you will naturally want to continue, because you feel better and better with each week!

By choosing to keep our bodies balanced with healthy food and consistent exercise, and our minds balanced with the right amount of mental relaxation and social stimulation, we decrease the stresses of life and this brings contentment and harmony. This true balance gives us peace of mind for not only a healthier, but a happier, more complete you!

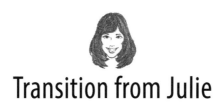

Transition from Julie

Transitioning...

When considering what advice I might provide about how to transition from 21 days to the rest of your life, I channeled Billy for a few moments...Billy is a bullet-list kind of guy, so here's me, being Billy:

1. Stick with Whole Foods!!!

If you stick with mostly whole foods you:

- Reduce unhealthy fats
- Reduce sugar
- Reduce calories
- Increase fiber
- Increase nutrition
- Increase Life Force

Ok, that last one was me and I have to be me...

Love Your Body
(Sounds Easy...Is Hard...Requires Practice)

If you've ever been married then you know that a healthy relationship is all about compromise and thinking about the other person first, before saying and doing things you might regret. It's the same with your body.

If you love pasta or pizza, compromise and eat it once a week. Without compromise, it's impossible to have a healthy relationship with your body.

Think before you eat! Ask yourself, "**Where is the love?**" Is the food you're about to consume food that you would offer to someone you love? Whether or not you're a fan of the *Black Eyed Peas*, in four short words, their lyric makes an awesome mantra!

Having a great mantra is an essential part of the health maintenance I teach all my clients. We like to think that other people are so "together," but it's just not so. We all have good days and less-good days. The difference between people who are successful in maintaining healthy habits, even under times of stress, even extreme stress, and those who fall off the cliff in those same circumstances, is in the systems they have in place to support themselves. In my practice I call it, "**ECM**": Expectations—Core—Mantra.

1. **Define Expectations**
    - How many times per week do I want to eat out?
    - Where will my other food come from?
    - What is my fallback option?
        – Is it in my pantry?
        – Do I re-stock it regularly?
        – Am I on the lookout for new fallback meals?

2. **Build Your Core**
    - What do I do, once a week, no matter what?
    - Who supports me in this?

3. **Have a Mantra**
    - How do I keep myself on track?
    - What do I say to myself?

Defining your expectations is also called planning. Without doing so, you set yourself up for failure and risk feeling down on yourself.

Building your core is how I refer to exercise, which includes all body movement and physical practices. Okay, Billy has told you to do it more than once a week, and truly, once a week is not ideal, but if you feel like the walls are falling down around you, make sure there is one activity you are going to do every single week, no matter what!

It can be a yoga practice, a strength-training session or a long walk. By having someone else involved in your core activity, be it a friend who walks with you, a trainer or instructor, or a family member who calls you out if you stop, the support makes persevering easier. If you stick with your core in tough times, you'll get right back on track when things ease up—because if you stuck to it once a week, you never STOPPED!!!

A few years ago, I rode the chair lift as a "single" to the top of *Elk Mountain*, in Pennsylvania, with an eighty-two-year-old man. Yes, I asked him how old he was.

Then I asked him what he eats for breakfast because I ask this question of every healthy older person I meet (the answer was oats). The man was born and raised in Switzerland. "You're still skiing," I said to him. "That's awesome!" He responded, "When I was a child, at recess the teachers would open up the classroom doors, point to the mountain and tell us to run up. So every day I ran up the mountain...and I just **NEVER STOPPED!**"

A **mantra** is a word or short phrase (4–5 words) that you can repeat to yourself. It can be simple like, "I can do this!" My son, Daniel, uses the one from the *Anger Management* movie, "Goosfraba." Lately, I've been using, "Keep your heart up," 4 sage words from my mom...Thanks, Mom!

Find one that resonates with you. That goes for the food as well. If something doesn't work well for you, don't eat it. Just because avocadoes are a good food for some people doesn't mean they're good for you! Your body is unique and individual, so tune out the noise, listen to your body and eat the whole foods that fuel you best...and just **NEVER STOP!**

Appendix A:
Exercises

BALL SQUATS

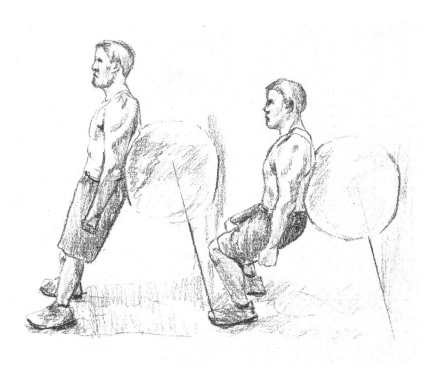

Start Position   **Finish Position**

Place ball behind lower back against wall, slowly lower yourself (4 seconds) and squat down so knees are almost at a 90-degree angle. Press up through heels; roll back up to starting position. *Note when you squat down, knees should be behind toes.

15 to 20 repetitions

PUSHUPS (MODIFIED)

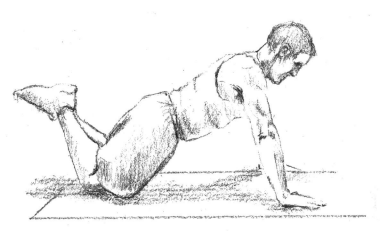

Start Position

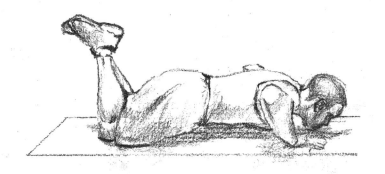

Finish Position

From your knees, place hands shoulder-width apart and with chest a few inches from the floor, push up until arms are straight. Try not to hike hips up, keeping back nice and straight. Return slowly to starting position. **Other great alternative start-up pushups:** Do pushups against a wall with your feet about 2 feet away from the wall or do pushups on stairs, starting on about the 4th step and gradually advance to the next step down as you get stronger!

15 to 20 repetitions

PUSHUPS

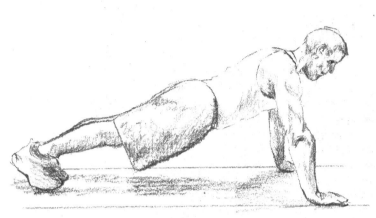

Start Position

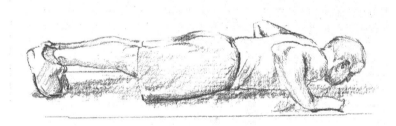

Finish Position

Place hands shoulder-width apart and chest a few inches from the floor, keeping back straight, push up until arms are straight. Return slowly to starting position. Be sure to keep your abdominals tight and do not hike hips up or allow hips to sag down.

15 to 20 repetitions

LAT PULLDOWNS (BAND)

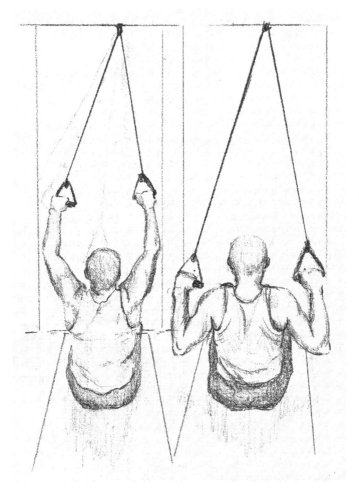

Start Position   **Finish Position**

Shut exercise band door with anchor in top of doorway. While sitting or kneeling on the floor, lean back slightly, with hands slightly wider than shoulder width, pull band down to upper chest. Return slowly in 4 seconds to starting position.

15 to 20 repetitions

LUNGES

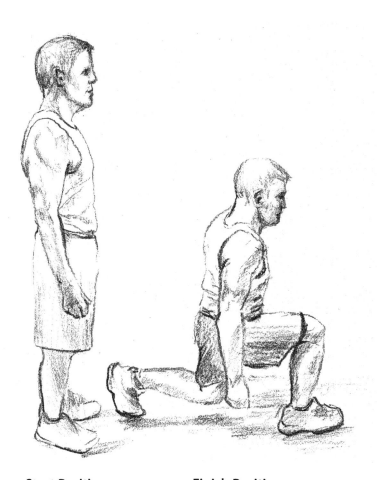

Start Position   **Finish Position**

With legs shoulder-width apart, head up, back straight, lunge forward in a wide stride, bending both legs simultaneously until forward thigh is parallel to the floor. Push back through forward foot and return slowly to starting position. Do all repetitions to one side and then repeat on the other side. *Safety note: When lunging forward, be sure to keep your forward knee behind your front foot.

15 to 20 repetitions

CHEST PRESS (BAND)

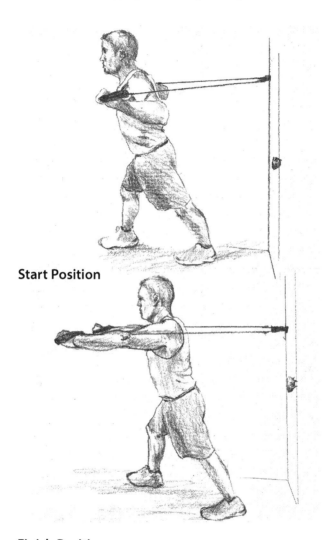

Start Position

Finish Position

Attach exercise band with anchor in closed door at chest level. With staggered stance, and arms slightly wider than shoulder width, fully extend arms straight out in front of you. Return slowly in 4 seconds back to starting position.

15 to 20 repetitions

SEATED ROW (BAND)

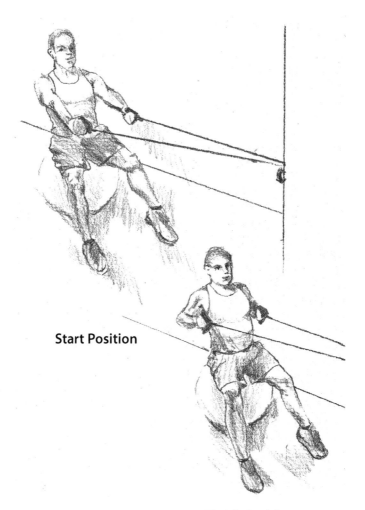

Start Position

Finish Position

Attach exercise band around a pole or with door anchor in closed door at chest level. Sitting on ball, torso erect, pull band back past rib cage, bringing chest out and shoulder blades pinched back. Return arms slowly in 4 seconds back to starting position.

15 to 20 repetitions

STEP-UPS

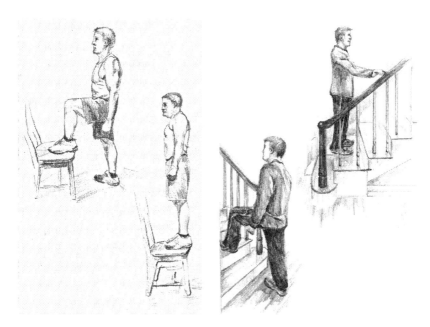

Start Position   Finish Position   Start Position   Finish Position

With head up, back straight, step one foot up on **sturdy knee-high** bench or chair, return slowly back to starting position. Do all repetitions on one side and then repeat on the other side. A great alternative is to do step-ups on your stairs. Step same as above but step up to the second step. For balance and support, hold the railing.

15 to 20 repetitions

PLANK

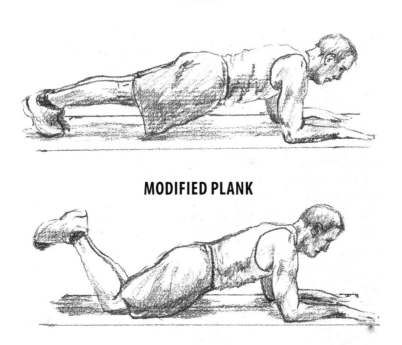

MODIFIED PLANK

Modified: Lie face down, rise up onto elbows and knees, keeping hips up, abdominals tight and back straight. Hold for 15-60 seconds.

LEG-ARM LIFT

Start Position

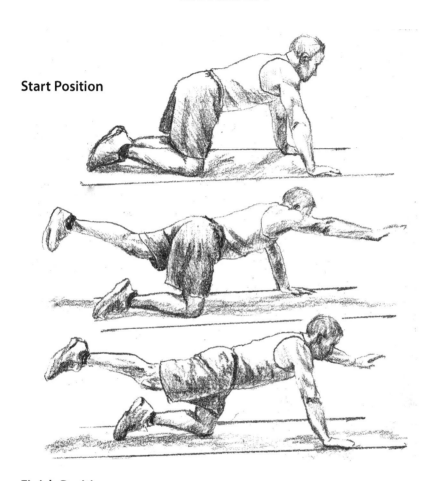

Finish Position

From all fours, extend opposite arm and leg as straight as possible, hold for 5 seconds. Return slowly to starting position. Alternate reps on opposite side.

15 to 20 repetitions

(Begin on Week 2)
BALL ABDOMINAL OBLIQUE CURL

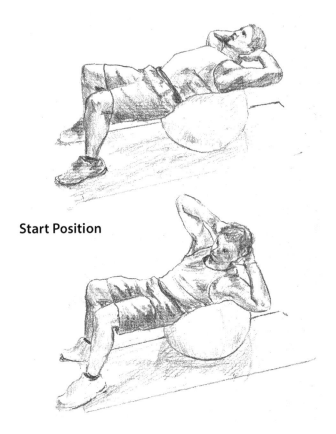

Start Position

Finish Position

Lying on the large exercise ball positioned midway on your back, hands behind your head and elbows wide, tighten abdominals, curl slowly up, raising shoulders and upper back off ball. Twist up, bringing elbow up and across towards opposite knee. Then pause at top, keeping head and neck in line with spine. Keep lower back balanced on ball. Return slowly back for 4 seconds to starting position. Perform alternate reps to opposite side, returning slowly to starting position between reps.

15 to 20 repetitions

BALL ABDOMINAL CURL

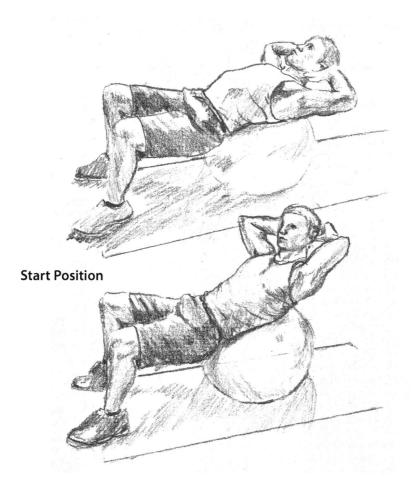

Start Position

Finish Position

Lying on the large exercise ball midway on your back, hands behind your head and elbows wide, tighten abdominals, curl slowly forward, raising shoulders and upper back forward when coming off ball. Pause at top. Keep head and neck in line with spine. Keep lower back on ball. Return slowly back for 4 seconds to starting position.

15 to 20 repetitions

(Begin on Week 3)
BICEP CURL (BAND)

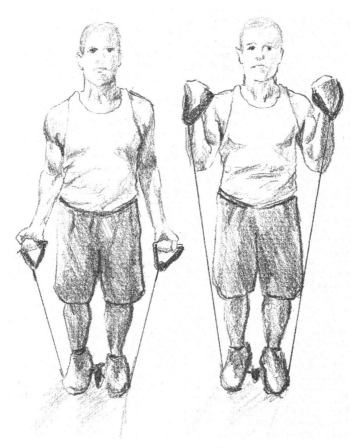

Start Position   **Finish Position**

Stand on medium band, knees slightly bent, hold handles at side, palms in. Curl arms towards shoulders, rotating palms up while curling arms up. Hold for 2 seconds and then return slowly in 4 seconds back to starting position.

15 to 20 repetitions

(Begin on Week 3)
CHEST FLY (BAND)

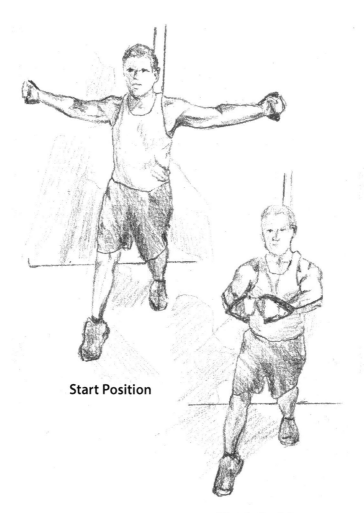

Start Position

Finish Position

Start with arms wide, elbows slightly bent, cross arms just past midline of body under lower chest, touch fists together, keeping elbows and knees slightly bent. Return slowly back in 4 seconds to starting position.

15 to 20 repetitions

(Begin on Week 2)
HIP "ABDUCTION"

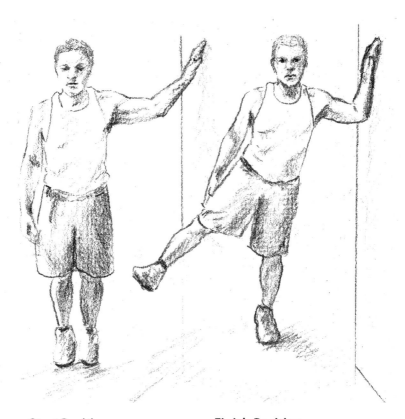

Start Position   **Finish Position**

Stand, holding support, flex foot up and "abduct" leg straight outward, away from body. Hold for 2 seconds away from body then slowly return in 4 seconds back to starting position. Do all reps on same leg, then switch legs and repeat.

15 to 20 repetitions

(Begin on Week 2)
OVERHEAD PRESS (BAND)

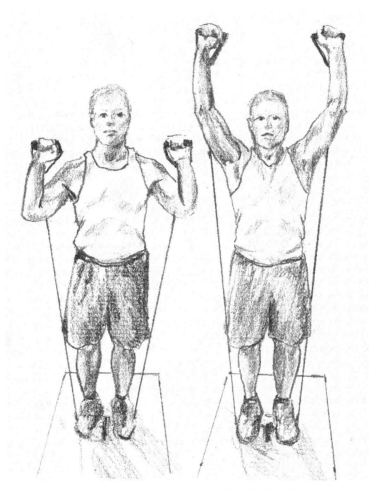

Start Position   **Finish Position**

Stand on light-weight band and with hands at shoulder-width, knees slightly bent, extend arms and press handles up overhead. Return slowly in 4 seconds to your shoulders.

15 to 20 repetitions

Appendix B: Stretches

HAMSTRING STRETCH

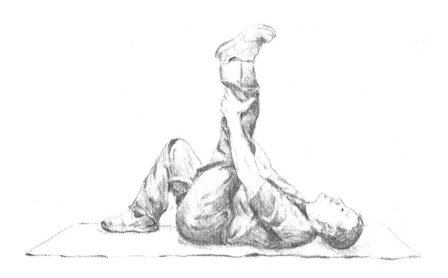

Hamstring

Lying on your back, with right knee bent and foot flat on the floor, extend your left leg straight up while keeping a slight bend in the knee. Hold your lower leg by the calf and pull leg towards your head. Hold stretch for 30 to 60 seconds and then switch legs. *Muscles stretched: Hamstring and Calf*

HIP AND GLUTE STRETCH

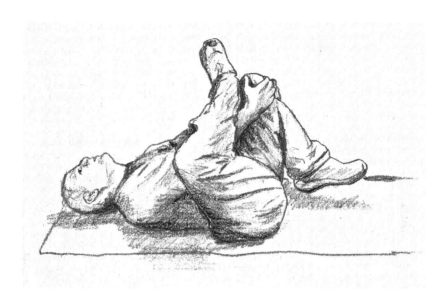

Hip & Glute

Lie on your back, with both knees bent and feet flat, then cross right foot over left knee at ankle, reach hands through and under right leg and around left knee, pull left knee towards your chest. Hold 30 to 60 seconds then switch legs. *Muscles stretched: Hip and Glute*

COBRA STRETCH

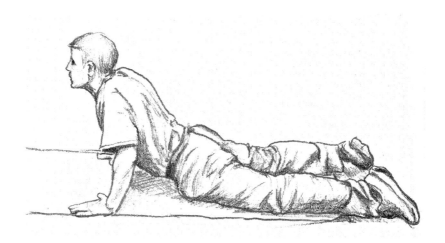

Cobra (back extension)

Lie face-down, keeping your hips on the floor. Place your hands beneath you, positioned slightly wider than your shoulders at chest level, curl your shoulders back first then press your upper body off the floor, keeping your hips on the floor. Hold for 30 to 60 seconds. Repeat few more times if you'd like. *Muscles stretched: Abdominals, Chest, Shoulders, Hip Flexors (psoas)*

CHILD'S POSE STRETCH

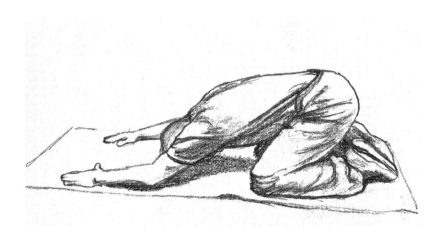

Child's Pose

From on all-fours, sit your buttocks back towards your heels. Allow your knees to go wider than your shoulders. Bring your head towards the floor and extend your arms straight out overhead and slide hands on the floor, keeping your glutes close to your heels. Hold for 30 to 60 seconds. *Muscles stretched: Low back, Shoulders, Mid-back*

HIP FLEXOR STRETCH

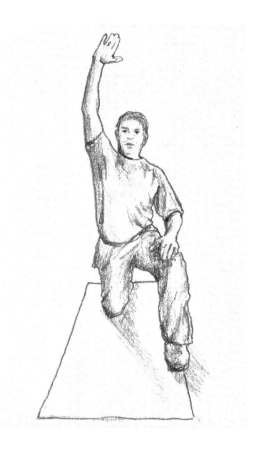

Hip Flexor

Start on knees then place left foot up flat on ground with left knee bent. Extend your right arm as high as you can overhead, extend your chest out and lean back slightly. Balance yourself by placing your left hand on your left thigh. Hold stretch for 30 to 60 seconds. Switch legs. *Muscles stretched: Hip flexors (psoas), Chest, Shoulders*

DOORWAY CHEST STRETCH

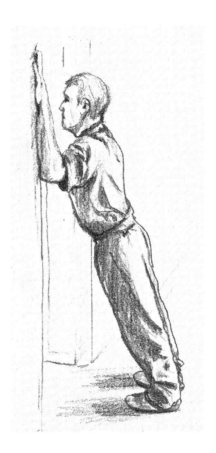

Doorway Stretch

Stand 6 to 12 inches away from an open doorway. Place forearms and hands on the doorway frame. Keep your feet flat and heels down. Slowly ease your body into the doorway. Step farther away for a deeper stretch. Hold for 30 to 60 seconds. *Muscles stretched: Chest, Shoulders, Calf*

Appendix C: Recipes

Nut Chart

Nut	Number of Shelled Nuts per 1 oz. serving	Calories
Almonds	20 - 24	160
Brazil nuts	6 - 8	190
Cashews	16 - 18	160
Hazelnuts	18 - 20	180
Macadamias	10 - 12	200
Peanuts	28	170
Pecans	18 - 20 halves	200
Pine nuts (pignolias)	150 -157	160
Pistachios	45 - 47	160
Walnuts	14 halves	190

Basic Grains

There are many wonderful books and resources on how to cook grains. My basic methods for basmati rice, farro, kasha, and quinoa are included here since they are used in the sample meal ideas.

I am a proponent of soaking all grains that can be soaked, to reduce phytates, sometimes called "antinutrients," and make the grains more digestible. To soak or not to soak...over the years I have tried both ways. I have found that soaking grains gives them a more pleasing texture, irrespective of the "nutrition" benefits, which are perpetually debated. In addition, soaking rice can shorten the cooking time by 5 or 10 minutes which is always a bonus!

If you are buying frozen, pre-cooked, whole grains, you can contact the manufacturer to ask whether or not they soak their grains before cooking them.

As for inorganic arsenic in rice, a recent study showed that rinsing rice multiple times reduced inorganic arsenic levels in both types of basmati rice. Combining the rinsing with a higher water volume cooking method (6:1 ratio of water to rice) reduced inorganic arsenic levels even further.[6]

White basmati rice requires rinsing to eliminate excess starch so the rinsing is just business as usual. Typically after rinsing, however, white basmati is soaked and then cooked in less water since it absorbs some of the soaking water and rice is cooked primarily by steam. I cook white basmati in homemade stock and do not use the 6:1 liquid to rice ratio when cooking with stock. This is my preference, however, the same higher water volume cooking directions given for the brown basmati can be used to cook white basmati; the white rice just requires a shorter cooking time.

I use the same rinsing method described in the white basmati cooking directions for the brown basmati. Note that when you rinse brown basmati the water does not appear "cloudy" so just give it 4 to 6 good rinses. After rinsing, I soak brown basmati for 8 hours or overnight.

---

[6] Raab, A., C. Baskaran, J. Feldmann, and A. Meharg. 2008. "Cooking Rice in a High Water to Rice Ratio Reduces Inorganic Arsenic Content." *Journal of Environmental Monitoring*, 2009, 11, 41-44. © The Royal Society of Chemistry 2009

BASIC WHITE BASMATI RICE

Ingredients:
   1 cup white basmati rice
   1 ½ cups water or homemade stock

Directions:
1. Rinse the rice 4–6 times until the water appears clear. I have found the easiest way to do this is to put the rice in a large, fine-mesh strainer. Perch the strainer on top of a deep bowl so the handle overhangs the top of the bowl and the body of the strainer is inside the bowl. Place bowl in the sink and run water over the strainer, filling the bowl so the water is covering the rice. The first few times you do this the water will look very cloudy. Give the water and rice in the strainer a stir or two with a wooden spoon, then lift the strainer out and dump the water. Replace the strainer and rinse again, repeating until the water on top of the rice looks clear. Once it is clear, rinse out the bowl and place the strainer with rice back on top of the bowl, filling with water one more time. Let rice soak for at least a half hour and up to two hours. Sometimes I only soak the rice for 20 minutes—I don't sweat it! Discard soaking water and rinse one more time.

2. Bring water or stock to a boil in a covered pot. Add rice, cover and bring back to boil. Reduce heat and simmer, covered tightly, for about 20 minutes.

3. Remove pot from heat, let sit for a few minutes and fluff gently with fork.

Makes 3 cups of cooked rice

Variations:

- Add a tablespoon of butter or oil to pot and sauté rice, stirring constantly and "drying" grains before adding boiling water or stock.

- When making a flavored pilaf, sauté chopped onion or shallots in a tbsp. of butter or oil for a few minutes first, sprinkling with sea salt, then add rice and sauté a few additional minutes to dry and coat grains before adding boiling water or stock and any preferred seasonings.

BASIC BROWN BASMATI RICE

Ingredients:

1 cup brown basmati rice, soaked 8 hours or overnight

6 cups water

Directions:

1. The night before you want to cook your brown rice, follow the rinsing instructions in step 1 of the *Basic White Basmati Rice* directions on the previous page. Note that brown basmati will not make the water "cloudy" so just rinse the rice 4 to 6 times. After rinsing, place rice in a bowl and cover with an inch or two of fresh water. Let it soak overnight. I also add a squeeze of fresh lemon juice to the soaking water, as the acid helps mitigate the phytates in brown rice. Discard the soaking water and thoroughly rinse rice.

2. Bring 6 cups of water to a boil and add brown rice. Cover the pot and simmer gently for about 35 – 40 minutes or until desired doneness. Drain rice in fine mesh strainer and serve. **Note:** Be sure to simmer the rice gently or the starch will overflow all over your pot and stove burner!

BASIC FARRO

Farro is an ancient wheat grain cultivated in Italy. It is available in pearled, semi pearled and "whole" varieties. The pearled and semi pearled varieties cook faster because some or all of the outer bran has been polished off (taking some of the nutrients with it).

Determining which type of farro you're getting is a challenge I have repeatedly encountered, especially when buying it from a bulk bin, but I have also had the issue with packaged farro that was incorrectly labeled or not labeled at all. My solution is to always soak farro, regardless of which type I think I have.

Farro should always be rinsed but unlike white basmati rice, you don't need to rinse it repeatedly; just give it one good rinse and place it in a bowl to soak overnight. I also add a squeeze of lemon juice to the soaking water.

Farro cooks by boiling so you don't have to worry about the amount of cooking water you're using unless you're trying to cook it like risotto, in which case you can just keep adding more hot water or stock, as it is absorbed, until you get a soft, creamy consistency. This will require a longer cooking time.

Ingredients:

1 cup farro, rinsed, soaked and drained and rinsed again.

4 cups of water

Directions:

1. Bring water to a boil.

2. Add farro, cover and reduce heat to simmer. Cook for 20 to 25 minutes or until desired tenderness. Taste the farro for texture to determine if it is ready. It is a chewy grain, but it should not be hard. Whole farro takes longer to cook so you need to taste and test. Drain excess water when cooking is complete.

Makes about 3 cups of cooked grain

Variations:

- Farro can be cooked in stock, like rice. If you want to cook it in stock, try using a 3:1 ratio of stock to farro, adding more hot stock if the farro isn't tender enough and all the stock is absorbed.

- When cooking is complete, adding a tablespoon of olive oil will keep the farro from sticking together.

- Farro is a great grain to freeze. Cook extra and freeze in single serving size portions.

- Cooked farro will last in the fridge for 4 days.

- Try adding cooked farro to your green salad or using it for breakfast porridge.

Note: Farro is a type of wheat and contains gluten. It is not suitable for anyone requiring a gluten-free diet.

BASIC KASHA

Kasha is buckwheat; actually, it is toasted buckwheat groats. Ironically, buckwheat isn't wheat at all, it's related to rhubarb and it is gluten free!

If you have Eastern European roots, you may have eaten it in a dish called "Kasha Varnishkes" made with onion, egg, and bowtie pasta.

Kasha cooks quickly, in 20 minutes tops, the same amount of time as white rice, quinoa and soaked pearled farro, making it a convenient whole grain.

I sometimes use cooked kasha as a substitute for bread crumbs, as in the turkey meatloaf recipe on page 191, or as a hearty winter breakfast porridge. When I eat kasha in the morning, I feel as if I can walk the frigid tundra for hours before getting hungry again!

Ingredients:

1 cup kasha—no rinsing or soaking required!

2 cups of water

½ tsp. sea salt

Directions:

1. Bring water to a boil and add sea salt.

2. Add kasha to boiling water, cover and reduce heat to low simmer.

3. Simmer, covered, for about 18–20 minutes until kasha is cooked and water is absorbed. Fluff with fork before serving.

Note: Kasha can be cooked in stock, with or without added fats and sautéed with chopped vegetables for a pilaf.

BASIC QUINOA

Quinoa gets a lot of publicity these days for being the only "grain" (botanically it is a seed) that is a "complete" protein, meaning that it has all the essential amino acids (essential means we need to get them from our diet).

What I love the most about quinoa is that it cooks so fast! It cooks in the same amount of time as white rice but has so much more to offer.

The recipe for Greek Quinoa Salad on page 194 outlines the basic cooking method for quinoa. Use a 2:1 ratio of water to quinoa. Quinoa is rinsed but not soaked. Dry toasting the grain is optional, but adding dryer grain to water that is already boiling results in a fluffier pilaf with less sticky grains. It is my preferred method unless I'm super short on time or I'm cooking it specifically for porridge.

If you've never tried quinoa and you'd like to introduce it gradually, try creating a grain pilaf by mixing ½ cup quinoa with 1 cup white basmati rice. They have approximately the same cooking times and cook well together. You can dry toast the grains together, remove grains and add water (use 2 ½ cups), bringing it to a boil before adding the grains back in.

Once the 2:1, rice to quinoa ratio is hardly noticeable to your palate, try making the pilaf with half rice and half quinoa before jumping into 100% quinoa dishes. Even if you love the taste of quinoa, making mixed grain pilafs provides flavor variety.

POACHED EGGS

Cook's Notes:

- If you've never tried poached eggs, you're in for a treat! Poaching eggs keeps the yolk soft and "runny," making a scrumptious "icing" for the foods eaten with your eggs.

- From a health perspective, poached eggs are hard to beat; since water boils at 220° F., cooking the eggs this way prevents the cholesterol in the yolk from oxidizing and you don't have to heat any added fats to cook the eggs, a win/win combination!

Ingredients:

Eggs

Water

Splash of vinegar

Directions:

1. Bring a small pot of water to a boil (2 qt. pot is big enough to poach 2 or 3 eggs).

2. Add a splash of apple cider or white vinegar to pot (you don't have to measure...the vinegar is just to help keep the egg together).

3. Break each of your eggs into a small cup (I use tea cups with handles). When water is boiling, hold cup near top of water and gently roll egg into boiling water—do this with both cups and immediately start timer for 3 minutes.

4. When timer goes off, remove eggs quickly with a slotted spoon to drain excess water, and gently place eggs on plate or plop directly onto greens, grain or toast!

GRAB & GO OVERNIGHT OATS

By Fara Cohen

Cook's Notes:

- There are many variations of this old-fashioned method of "soaking" oats instead of cooking them. Recently, many oat recipes have appeared on the net using mason jars, but any covered pint-sized container works. The mason jars have a pleasing, "artsy" look to them and eating the "whole jar" feels decadent—a bit like a cupcake, only mushier!

- The basic "formula" is a 2:1 ratio of "liquid" to oats, adding flavorings and textures to taste. For thicker cereal use half yogurt and half milk.

- Put dried fruit in the night before or add berries or fresh fruit in the morning. If you need crunch, try adding chopped apple or 1-2 tbsp. of sliced almonds.

- Even though it's "Grab & Go," sit down to eat it!

Ingredients:

½ cup old-fashioned oats (not instant or steel cut)

½ cup unsweetened almond milk (or dairy milk)

½ cup plain yogurt

2 tbsp. apple juice-sweetened dried cranberries

¼ tsp. vanilla

1 tsp. real maple syrup

Tiny pinch of sea salt

Generous sprinkling of cinnamon

Directions:

Put all ingredients in a jar or other one-pint container and stir to mix well. Cover container and put in fridge overnight. Can store up to 2 days before eating.

JULIE'S (CHICKEN) FRIED RICE

Ingredients:
1 tbsp. extra-virgin olive oil

1 tbsp. butter (preferably grass-fed)

1 to 2 cloves garlic, peeled and minced

1 onion, chopped

1 egg, beaten

Tamari or Shoyu (soy sauce) to taste

Gomasio or toasted sesame seeds

About 4 scallions, sliced

2 cups leftover rice

1 to 2 cups diced leftover chicken—optional

Directions:
1. Heat the olive oil in a large skillet. Add onion and sauté for 3–4 minutes. Add garlic and sauté one more minute.

2. Gather onion and garlic to center of pan, place butter on top and pour beaten egg over melted butter. Scramble egg into small pieces with spatula.

3. Add the leftover rice (and meat, if using) to the pan, mixing it in with onions and egg mixture and seasoning it to taste with soy sauce and gomasio (or toasted sesame seeds).

4. When heated through, sprinkle scallions on top and serve.

Serves 4 as a side, 2 as a main course

Sesame seeds can be toasted on a baking sheet in a 350° F. oven for 8–10 minutes. Careful not to burn! They can also be toasted in a dry skillet over medium to low heat; remove when seeds smell toasty and begin to turn a golden color – be super careful not to burn.

ROASTED SWEET POTATO WEDGES (aka SWEET POTATO FRIES)

Cook's Notes:

- I like to use chili powder, cinnamon and salt to season yams but feel free to use any seasonings you enjoy (olive oil, rosemary and sea salt are also delicious!)

Ingredients:

Yams (any variety you enjoy, preferably organic)

Coconut oil

Chili powder

Cinnamon

Sea salt

Directions:

1. Pre-heat oven to 375 degrees F.

2. Scrub potatoes with brush to clean thoroughly.

3. Leave skin on, and cut potatoes, first in half by length, then in half by width. Place flat side of cut potato against cutting board and slice into 4 quarters or 6-8 smaller "wedges," depending on size of potato. Thinner wedges cook faster.

4. Place rimmed baking sheet in pre-heated oven for 3–4 minutes. Remove hot baking sheet carefully and plop a tablespoon or two of coconut oil onto the sheet (use about 1-2 tbsp. oil per pound of potatoes). When the oil is melted, place potato wedges on sheet and mix thoroughly to coat with oil. Spread potatoes into one layer with no overlaps. Sprinkle lightly with chili powder—this you don't need to measure! Then sprinkle with cinnamon. Lastly, sprinkle lightly with sea salt.

5. Bake for about 40 minutes or until desired crispness is reached. Be careful not to overcook as they can turn to charcoal rather fast!

Serving size is 1–1 ½ cups of wedges

MEDITERRANEAN SPAGHETTI SQUASH

Adapted from a recipe by Leah Hatley

Cook's Notes:

- *Muir Glen®* Brand fire roasted diced tomatoes are delicious when tomatoes are out of season.

- Fresh basil makes a big difference in this recipe—buy fresh instead of using dried, if possible.

- Cooking time varies based on the size of squash and your oven temperature (35–50 minutes).

- Little kids are fascinated by the strands of "spaghetti" that can be scooped out of the cooked squash...let them help if you have time...children are much more invested in eating foods they have helped to prepare.

Ingredients:

2 spaghetti squash, halved lengthwise and seeded

2 tbsp. extra virgin olive oil plus extra for brushing

1 onion, chopped

2 cloves garlic, minced

1 ½ cups chopped tomato or 1 to 2 14.5 oz. cans of diced tomatoes, liquid drained

½ cup crumbled feta cheese

½ tsp. oregano

2 tbsp. chopped fresh basil (or 2 tsp. dried) or more to taste (I use about 1 cup of loosely packed fresh basil)

Sea salt and fresh black pepper

Directions:

1. Preheat oven to 375° F.

2. Cut spaghetti squash in half, length-wise, and scoop out seeds. Brush halves with extra virgin olive oil and place spaghetti squash, flesh sides down, on a baking sheet. Bake 40 minutes or until a fork can be inserted with only a little resistance. Remove squash from oven, and set aside to cool enough to be easily handled.

3. Meanwhile, heat olive oil in a skillet over medium low heat. Sauté onion until tender, sprinkling with pinch of sea salt. Add garlic and sauté for 1 to 2 more minutes. Stir in the tomatoes. Add oregano (and basil if using dried) and cook only until tomatoes are warm. Remove from heat and add the (fresh) basil and feta cheese.

4. Use a fork to scoop the stringy pulp (a.k.a. "spaghetti") from the squash, and place in a medium bowl. Toss with the sautéed vegetable mixture. Taste for seasoning, adding sea salt and/or fresh black pepper to taste. Serve warm.

This recipe makes delicious leftovers which you can use as a lunchtime "Main Course" (see sample lunch ideas for cookers). Serving Size (for adults) is about 2 cups, which is about half of an average-size spaghetti squash.

Recipe makes 4 servings

FARRO SALAD

Cook's Notes:

- This salad doesn't need salt as the olives are savory and the Zatar also contains salt.
- If you don't have Zatar try substituting ½ tsp. of cumin and taste before adding salt.
- If you're not a fan of olives, try a few marinated sun-dried tomatoes, chopped.
- Farro also tastes delicious mixed into a green salad with your favorite salad veggies and dressing.

Ingredients:

¾ cup cooked farro (leftover)

5 pitted Kalamata olives, chopped

½ of an apple, cored (skin on) and chopped

2 tbsp. feta cheese

Dressing:

1 tbsp. extra virgin olive oil

1 tbsp. red wine vinegar

½ tsp. Zatar (available from Penzeys.com)

Freshly ground pepper to taste

Directions:

1. Mix farro, chopped olives, apple and feta cheese in a bowl. Add all dressing ingredients to small jar and shake well. Pour dressing over farro salad, mix well and taste for seasoning.

2. Enjoy!

1 Serving

ITALIAN-STYLE GREEN BEANS

by Ann Marie Giraldi

Ingredients:

1 lb. green beans

¼ of red onion, thinly sliced

5 grape tomatoes, sliced in half

1 tbsp. good quality extra virgin olive oil

Sea salt to taste—I use about ¼ tsp. sea salt for 1 lb. of green beans.

Directions:

1. Cook beans in boiling water, with a pinch of sea salt added, for about 5-6 minutes until cooked well but still crisp.

2. Drain beans in colander and add ice to stop cooking.

3. Toss beans with onion and tomato. Add olive oil and mix until beans look "shiny." Place on a platter and sprinkle with sea salt to taste.

Makes 3½ to 4, generous one-cup servings

GREEN BEAN AND ARUGULA SALAD

For variety, toss a few cups of arugula or baby arugula with warm, cooked and dressed green beans like the Italian-Style Green Beans above. The warm beans will slightly wilt the arugula and the olive oil and salt on the beans will provide all the "dressing" you need. I really love this combination and it's so easy!

PESTO TOMATO BOWL

Ingredients:

1 cup cherry tomatoes (sliced in half)

¼ cup blanched and sliced almonds

¼ cup feta cheese

1 tbsp. prepared pesto or 1 tbsp. pesto paste mixed with 1 tbsp. warm water.

Directions:

Wash and slice cherry tomatoes. Add almonds and feta cheese and stir. Pour pesto over tomato bowl and stir gently to mix. Enjoy!

Serves 1

TUNA WHITE BEAN SALAD

Adapted from a recipe from Ann Marie

Cook's Notes:

- If you are using tuna packed in water, add 1 tablespoon of extra virgin olive oil to the Ponzu and mustard. Albacore tuna packed in extra virgin olive oil tastes best for this recipe.

- Use leftover beans in salads or with grains. Beans last for 4 days in the fridge, but don't store in metal can.

Ingredients:

1 whole fire-roasted red pepper, chopped

2 Hearts of Palm (about 4 inches long each), chopped

1, 5 ounce can wild albacore tuna in olive oil, not drained

1 cup of cannellini beans, rinsed and drained

1 tbsp. Ponzu sauce

1 tsp. Dijon mustard

¼ tsp. sea salt

Freshly ground black pepper to taste

Sprinkling of red chili flakes

Directions:

1. Combine chopped pepper, hearts of palm and beans in mixing bowl. Open tuna (pull-top lids are extremely sharp!) and empty the tuna with olive oil (do not drain) into the mixing bowl with beans and veggies. Sprinkle with ¼ tsp. of sea salt and fresh pepper to taste and mix thoroughly.

2. In a ramekin or small jar, mix 1 tbsp. Ponzu sauce and one teaspoon of mustard. Pour sauce over bean and tuna mixture and mix. Sprinkle with red chili flakes and freshly ground black pepper to taste. This salad needs some time for the flavors to blend – refrigerate for 20 minutes for best taste.

Serves 2

CHICKEN LETTUCE WRAPS WITH PEANUT SAUCE

Cook's Notes:

- Breast meat or a combination of white and dark meat from leftover rotisserie chicken works equally well.

- If you're brown-bagging this, put a toothpick in your wrap to hold it closed and place in a sturdy container, or transport components separately and assemble on site.

Ingredients:

1 cup leftover chicken, diced or in small strips

Iceberg or Butter lettuce leaves—3 large outer leaves

3 scallions, white part and one-inch of green, thinly sliced

Directions:

1. Carefully remove and rinse lettuce leaves.

2. Gently place 1/3 cup of chicken in center of leaf and sprinkle 1/3 of scallions on top.

3. Pour one tbsp. of Peanut Sauce over chicken, gently roll leaf, and enjoy! Rinse, repeat...

Peanut Sauce Ingredients:

2 tbsp. creamy (smooth) peanut butter

½ tbsp. shoyu or tamari soy sauce

¼ tsp. maple syrup

½ tsp. (heaping) grated fresh ginger (1-inch piece of fresh ginger, peeled and grated on microplane)

1 ½ tbsp. very warm water

Directions:

Add all ingredients to small jar or shaker bottle and mix thoroughly. If sauce is too thick, add a little more warm water.

Serves 1

BAKED COD, ITALIAN STYLE

Ingredients:
¾ lb. cod filet

1 small onion, thinly sliced

1 small zucchini, sliced into 1"-thick rounds

¾ tsp. basil

¼ tsp. granulated garlic powder

1 tbsp. capers

1, 8 oz. can tomato sauce

1, 14 oz. can diced tomatoes with ¼ cup of the juice (*Muir Glen®* organic fire-roasted diced tomatoes are delicious in this)

Sea salt and freshly ground pepper

Directions:
1. Preheat oven to 350° F.

2. Rinse and dry fish filet. Sprinkle both sides of fish with sea salt and fresh pepper.

3. Place the fish filet in an ungreased 9x13 glass baking dish. Mound the sliced onion and zucchini around the fish. Sprinkle the basil, garlic and capers over the fish and vegetables. Pour the tomato sauce and diced tomatoes with ¼ cup of juice over the top.

4. Bake for 45-60 minutes or until the fish is white and flakes easily (cod should always be thoroughly cooked). Baste the fish, once or twice, with the pan juices during baking.

Serves 2

ROASTED PORK TENDERLOIN WITH ONION & APPLES

Ingredients:
1 pork tenderloin (approx. 1 lb.)

2 apples, peeled, cored and sliced

1 medium onion, sliced

2 tbsp. extra virgin olive oil

1 cup water

½ cup organic shoyu or tamari (wheat-free) soy sauce

Directions:
1. Preheat oven to 400° F. Place rack in center of oven. Place dutch oven or enamel cast iron pot in oven to preheat.

2. Place clean, dry pork tenderloin into preheated pot and place pork, uncovered, in oven for 7 minutes per side (remove pan and turn meat over after first side has cooked for 7 minutes).

3. After pork has cooked for 14 minutes, remove pot with pork and lower oven temperature to 350°F. Put all remaining ingredients into pot and cover tightly.

4. Roast, covered for 60 minutes.

Serves 3 - 4

TURKEY MEATLOAF

Ingredients:

1 pound ground turkey (dark meat tastes best)

1 cup cooked kasha

3 cups (½ of a 5 oz. clamshell package) of baby spinach, chopped

½ medium onion, finely chopped

1 large carrot, finely chopped or grated

1-2 cloves garlic, minced

1 tsp. sea salt

1 tsp. favorite spice (Penzeys' brand Mural of Flavor is a delicious salt-free mix, or you can try chili powder)

1 egg

Directions:

1.   Preheat oven to 375° F. Place rack in center of oven.

2.   If you have a food processor, it's an easy way to grate carrots and chop spinach and onion.

3.   Mix all ingredients well and mold into loaf shape on jelly roll pan or baking dish.

4.   Roast, uncovered for 1 hour.

5.   Enjoy meatloaf with some harissa, sriracha or other hot sauce, if desired.

Serves 4

BLACK BEAN PATTIES
Adapted from a recipe from Catherine Kaczmarek

Ingredients:
1 can (15 oz.) of black beans, rinsed, drained and chopped

½ onion, chopped

¼ tsp. granulated garlic

2 tsp. Amore® brand chili pepper paste

1 tsp. cumin

¼ cup old-fashioned rolled oats

½ tsp. sea salt

Organic grits for dusting (an exception to the flour rule...to help crisp up these patties!)

2 tbsp. organic canola or safflower oil for cooking

Directions:
1. Cut onion into quarters and add to mini chopper. Chop onion and add to mixing bowl.

2. Add ½ the beans to mini chopper and chop until beans in bottom of chopper turn to paste. Add chopped beans to mixing bowl and repeat with remaining beans. **Note:** If you have a full-size food processor, you can add the onion and beans together and pulse until onions and beans form a thick paste.

3. Remove to mixing bowl; add cumin, garlic, salt and hot pepper paste and mix. Add oats and mix again.

4. Wet your hands and form batter into 4 cakes approximately 3 inches in diameter. Spread grits on a sheet of wax paper and place cakes on grits, turning to coat both sides.

5. Pan fry on stove top until warmed through and slightly crispy on outside. About 3–4 minutes per side. Patties are soft; for best results, wait for one side to get fairly crisp before flipping.

Serves 2 (2 cakes each)

SKIRT STEAK WITH CHIMICHURRI

by Peter Berley – www.peterberley.com

Cook's Notes:

- I use twice as much parsley as cilantro because I have a little of the "soap gene" for cilantro (cilantro tastes a bit like soap to some people). If you love cilantro, this is also delicious with a 1:1 ratio; adjust the herb ratios to suit your palate.

- Chimichurri sauce makes everything taste better and it is coveted in my home for topping eggs the morning after...good luck having any left to do that!

Ingredients:

2 pounds skirt steak

1 shallot, peeled and chopped

1 cup tightly packed parsley leaves

½ cup tightly packed cilantro leaves

1 small jalapeno pepper, seeded and coarsely chopped

1 tsp. sea salt

¼ cup rice vinegar

¾ cup extra virgin olive oil

Directions:

1. Combine all ingredients except for steak and olive oil in a food processor and pulse to finely chop. Add oil slowly until well combined.

2. Combine the steak and about ½ chimichurri and marinate for one hour at room temperature or overnight in the fridge. Turn several times.

3. Remove the meat from the marinade and allow marinade to drip off. Grill or pan-sear 4 to 5 minutes per side. Allow the steak to rest for 5 minutes before slicing across the grain. Serve with remaining chimichurri sauce on side.

Serves 4-6

GREEK QUINOA SALAD

Ingredients:

½ cup uncooked quinoa

1 cup water

2 radishes, diced small (about ¼ cup)

½ cup cucumber, diced small

¼ cup finely chopped red onion

1 cup garbanzo beans (chick peas)

3 cups baby spinach (about ½ of 5 oz. clamshell)

½ cup crumbled feta cheese

Dressing:

Juice of one-half lemon

1 tbsp. red wine vinegar

2 tbsp. extra virgin olive oil

1 tsp. of Penzeys Greek Seasoning, soaked in ½ tbsp. water

Directions:

1. Rinse quinoa in a fine mesh strainer until no foam appears. Dry toast quinoa in pan until it smells slightly nutty and grain is dry (couple of minutes). Remove grain from pan, add 1 cup water to pan and bring to boil. Add quinoa to boiling water, lower heat to simmer, cover and cook for 18 minutes. Spread cooked quinoa out on rimmed baking sheet to cool.

2. In a medium bowl stir together cooled quinoa, cucumbers, radish, onion and chickpeas.

3. In a small jar or shaker bottle combine lemon juice, red wine vinegar, olive oil and Greek Seasoning (or ½ tsp. oregano and ½ tsp. sea salt) and shake to mix.

4. Divide spinach leaves between two plates and top each plate with half of quinoa salad and ¼ cup of feta cheese.

Serves 2

EASY BROWN RICE AND BEANS

Cook's Notes:

- Some natural markets carry frozen brown rice and beans packaged together. *Stahlbush Island Farms, Inc.* brand offers frozen grain and bean combinations. This is a quick option.

- There is an ever-increasing selection of frozen cooked grains like quinoa. Experiment with these other easy whole grain options for a healthy variety in your diet.

Ingredients:

1 cup cooked brown rice (frozen cooked brown rice is fine)

½ cup black beans, drained and rinsed (or substitute pinto)

2 tbsp. shredded cheddar or other shredded cheese

¼ cup prepared salsa

¼ Hass-type avocado (about ¼ cup), diced (optional)

Directions:

Heat the brown rice according to package instructions (microwave or stovetop). Mix brown rice with beans. Stir in prepared salsa to taste and heat slightly if salsa is cold. Top mixture with 2 tbsp. shredded cheese and diced avocado, if desired.

Serves 1

EASY BROWN RICE AND PEAS

Cook's Notes:

- Fresh chives are a delicious topping for this quick and easy rice dish...if you don't have any, try a tablespoon of finely chopped red onion.

Ingredients:

1 cup cooked brown rice (frozen brown rice works well)

2/3 cup frozen organic peas, defrosted (let sit for 10 – 15 minutes at room temperature)

½ tsp. sea salt

¼ tsp. cumin

¼ tsp. paprika

Pinch of granulated garlic

Juice of ½ lemon

2 – 3 tbsp. water

½ tbsp. extra virgin olive oil

1 tbsp. fresh chives, chopped – about 4-5 chives

Directions:

1. Pour 2 – 3 tbsp. of water into small saucepan and heat. Add rice and stir until rice is heated through – about 5 minutes for frozen brown rice. Add peas, sea salt, cumin, paprika, pinch of garlic, and lemon juice and stir to blend seasonings and cook peas – about 3 or 4 more minutes.

2. Meanwhile, rinse fresh chives and chop.

3. Turn off heat and stir in ½ tbsp. olive oil, mixing thoroughly.

4. Remove brown rice and peas to a bowl and sprinkle with fresh chives.

5. Eat and Enjoy!

Serves 1

PESTO RICE SALAD WITH EDAMAME & WALNUTS

Cook's Notes:

- *Amore*® brand pastes come in "toothpaste" type squeeze tubes. Their products have a long shelf life (45 days from opening) and some varieties are Non-GMO Project Verified. They are a convenient condiment for single people and families alike. The *Amore*® website lets you search for stores by zip code and their products are also available online.

Ingredients:

1 cup cooked brown rice or white basmati rice

½ cup frozen organic shelled edamame, cooked according to package directions (I boil mine for about 12-14 minutes)

8 walnut halves (½ oz.), finely chopped

2 tbsp. *Amore*® brand pesto paste

¼ cup warm water

Freshly ground black pepper to taste

Sprinkling of red chili flakes (optional)

Directions:

1. Add pesto paste to ¼ cup of water and stir to mix.

2. Mix together rice, edamame and chopped walnuts. Pour pesto sauce over mixture. Season to taste with freshly ground pepper and chili flakes, if desired.

Serves 1

GREEN CHICKEN SALAD

Cook's Notes:

- When cutting an avocado in half, leave the pit in place and use the half without the pit first. Wrap remaining half, with pit in place, tightly in plastic wrap and refrigerate. Use within two days. The pit will help keep the avocado "greener".

- If you are making this salad with the "leftover" half, reserve the pit and push it into the leftover chicken salad for storing in fridge – the pit will also keep your salad "greener".

- If you want to eat your chicken salad in a delicata squash "boat", see steps 1 and 2 in the recipe, *Mediterranean Spaghetti Squash*, for instructions on how to roast a squash. The procedure for roasting all squash is the same but cooking time varies based on the size of your squash. For a delicata squash, which has tender skin that you can eat, start checking for doneness after 30 minutes.

Ingredients:

1 cooked chicken breast (about 8 oz.), shredded or

2 cups of shredded leftover cooked chicken—(rotisserie chicken works well!)

1 "fat" carrot or 2 "skinny" carrots, grated

1 stalk of celery, diced

½ cup of diced cucumber (about 1/3 of a 7-inch cucumber)

¼ cup blanched and sliced almonds

Dressing:

½ Hass-type avocado (about 1/2 cup)

½ cup water

½ tbsp. lemon juice (juice from ¼ lemon)

½ tbsp. apple cider vinegar

½ tbsp. extra virgin olive oil

½ tbsp. raw honey

¼ tsp. granulated garlic powder

¼ tsp. sea salt

Directions:

1. Combine diced chicken, carrots, celery and cucumber. Sprinkle almonds on mixture and stir.

2. Combine all dressing ingredients and blend in blender or Vitamix®, for 1 to 2 minutes or until smooth.

3. Pour dressing over salad and mix.

Makes 2–3 servings

SUPER SALMON SALAD

by Andrea Beaman – www.andreabeaman.com

Ingredients:

1 can wild-caught sockeye salmon (7.5 oz)

½ small red onion, peeled and diced small

1 tablespoon minced parsley

1 celery stalk, diced

Baby mixed greens or hollowed-out vegetables for stuffing

Dressing:

2 ½ tablespoons extra virgin olive oil

1 teaspoon Dijon mustard

1 teaspoon honey

1 ½ tablespoon apple cider vinegar

Sea salt and pepper to taste

Directions:

1. Drain salmon and place in mixing bowl. Use potato masher to mash salmon into small bits. Crush small bones with your just-washed fingers and do not remove fish skin or bones. (These edible bones keep your bones healthy and you won't even know they are there.)

2. Combine salmon with diced red onion, celery, and parsley.

3. Whisk olive oil, mustard, honey, apple cider vinegar, sea salt and pepper (I use about ¼ tsp. sea salt for single recipe). Pour dressing over salmon and mix thoroughly. Lay salmon salad on a bed of baby greens or stuff into hollowed-out vegetable like tomato or bell pepper.

Serves 2

BASIC BALSAMIC VINAIGRETTE

Ingredients:
1/3 cup extra virgin olive oil

3 tbsp. balsamic vinegar

½ tbsp. real maple syrup

½ tsp. sea salt

Freshly ground pepper to taste

Directions:
Shake all ingredients together in shaker bottle or small glass jar with lid. Leftover dressing lasts 1 week in fridge.

....

SIMPLE TAHINI SAUCE

Ingredients:
½ cup tahini (sesame butter)

Squeeze of fresh lemon juice (about ½ of large lemon)

½ cup of warm water (gently heat water — do not boil)

¼ tsp. paprika

¼ tsp. granulated garlic powder

¼ tsp. sea salt

1/8 tsp. cayenne pepper

Directions:
Shake together in glass jar. Leftover dressing lasts for 1 week in fridge.

YOGURT SAUCE

Ingredients:

½ cup plain whole milk yogurt

Juice of ½ lemon

1 tsp. extra-virgin olive oil

1 tsp. raw honey

1 ½ tsp. Penzeys Greek Seasoning mix dissolved in one tablespoon of water (or try ½ tsp. sea salt and 1 tsp. Italian seasoning mix)

Directions:

1. Use teaspoon for olive oil first then honey—this way honey will come off the spoon cleanly!

2. Put all ingredients in blender or shaker jar and mix well.

3. Yields ¾ cup dressing

Makes 3, scant ¼ cup servings

ROASTED BRUSSELS SPROUTS

Ingredients:
Fresh Brussels sprouts (about a pound)

1-2 tbsp. extra virgin olive oil

Sea salt

Directions:
1. Pre-heat the oven to 375° F. and arrange a rack in the middle.

2. Add the olive oil and sea salt (2 big pinches) in a mixing bowl. Wash Brussels sprouts. Slice off brown stem end and remove any other leaves that are browning.

3. Toss cleaned and trimmed sprouts into mixing bowl with oil and salt and stir repeatedly until sprouts are slightly shiny from oil. Place on rimmed baking sheet and roast for 20-35 minutes. Check for preferred tenderness and remove when you like the texture...they should be pleasantly crunchy but not tough.

Note: Root vegetables like rutabaga, beets, etc. can be thinly sliced and tossed with oil, salt and desired seasonings to make crisp "chips." Baking time will vary based on thickness of slices and desired crispness.

ROASTED ASPARAGUS

Ingredients:
Fresh asparagus
1 tsp. Organic canola oil (for brushing pan)
Extra virgin Olive oil
Sea salt

Directions:
1. Pre-heat the oven to 375° F.
2. Snap off ends of asparagus (they naturally break in the right place) and discard. Wash asparagus and arrange on flat baking sheet or jelly roll pan that has been brushed with canola oil.
3. Roast for 5 – 10 minutes, depending on thickness of stalks.
4. Remove from oven and drizzle with extra virgin olive oil and sea salt. Eat and enjoy!

ROASTED KALE CHIPS

Ingredients:
Washed, spun and torn or cut kale leaves (discard kale stems)
Oil of choice
Sea salt
Sprinkle of seasoning like sea salt, garlic or chili powder

Directions:
1. Preheat oven to 350° F.
2. Toss kale leaves with oil and spread on rimmed baking sheet(s) in single layer. Sprinkle with seasonings and bake 10–15 minutes—watch carefully as leaves burn very quickly.

CRUNCHY CHICKPEAS

Ingredients:
2 15-ounce cans of Garbanzo beans, drained and rinsed

2 tbsp. extra virgin olive oil

2 tsp. Zatar (available from Penzeys.com)

½ tsp. sea salt

Directions:
1. Heat the oven to 375° F. and arrange a rack in the middle.

2. Dry chickpeas as much as possible and pick out any loose skins. I use the insert of my salad spinner to rinse beans, then drop insert into spinner and spin to dry. You can also blot them dry with toweling.

3. Place the olive oil, Zatar and sea salt in a large bowl and stir to combine. Add chickpeas and mix thoroughly until the beans look shiny and are coated with spice mixture.

4. Spread the chickpeas in an even layer on a rimmed baking sheet and bake until crisp, about 40 minutes (Caution, chickpeas "pop" when they are heated!)

Makes about 6, ½ cup servings or 12, ¼ cup servings

RICE PUDDING

Ingredients:

    2 cups cooked (leftover) rice

    1 cup almond milk (use dairy milk if desired)

    1 tbsp. maple syrup

    1 tsp. vanilla

    1 tbsp. butter (grass-fed)

    Generous sprinkle of cinnamon

    Pinch of sea salt

Directions:

Combine all ingredients in small saucepan and heat on stovetop for 5-7 minutes or until mixture has the desired creamy texture.

Makes four, ½ cup servings

Appendix D:
Heart Rate & RPE Charts

Target Heart Rate Chart

AGE	55%	60%	70%	80%	85%
15	19	21	24	27	29
20	18	20	23	27	28
25	18	19	23	26	28
30	17	19	22	25	27
35	17	19	22	25	26
40	17	18	21	24	26
45	16	18	20	23	25
50	16	17	20	23	24
55	15	17	19	22	23
60	15	16	19	21	23
65	14	16	18	21	22
70	14	15	18	20	21
75	13	15	17	19	21
80	13	14	16	19	20
85	12	14	16	18	19
90	11	13	15	17	18

1-10 Borg Rating of Perceived Exertion Scale

0	Rest
1	Really Easy
2	Easy
3	Moderate
4	Sort of Hard
5	Hard
6	
7	Really Hard
8	
9	Really, Really Hard
10	Maximum: 100% exertion

About the Authors

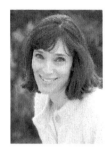 Julie Cohen is a Certified Holistic Health Counselor and founder of Mad Nutrition, LLC, which specializes in empowering people to upgrade their food choices and their lives.

From preparing healthier meals at home to learning how to make better food selections on the road, clients get the skills they need to attain their health and weight loss goals. Julie works with individuals from all over the country via internet coaching programs, as well as providing on site nutritional counseling and workshops in the New Jersey area.

To learn more about the services Julie offers please visit Mad Nutrition on the web at www.madnutrition.com.

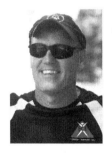 Bill McHugh is a Nationally Certified Personal Trainer and CEO of Fitness Coaching, Inc., a health and fitness management company that specializes in personalized wellness coaching to individuals, small groups and organizations.

Bill holds his Master's Degree in Fitness Management and has 25 years of comprehensive work in exercise prescription and health enhancement.

An engaging motivational speaker, Bill provides wellness seminars to corporations, hospitals and schools and delivers in-home and on-line private and group fitness training to all populations from the novice exerciser to elite athletes.

To learn more about the range of services Bill offers, please visit www.fitnesscoachinginc.com.

To join our conversation about living Balanced and Whole, visit us on the web at www.balancedandwhole.com.